MCQs for MRCOG Part 1

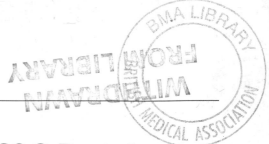

MCQs for MRCOG Part 1
A Self-assessment Guide

Richard de Courcy-Wheeler MD MRCOG
Consultant Obstetrician Gynaecologist
Daisy Hill Hospital, Newry
and
Honorary Clinical Lecturer, Department of Obstetrics and Gynaecology
Queen's University, Belfast, Northern Ireland

Bernie McElhinney MD MRCOG
Specialist Registrar
Royal Jubilee Maternity Service, Royal Maternity Hospital, Belfast,
Northern Ireland

Khaled El-Hayes MB BCh MS CABOG
Daisy Hill Hospital, Newry, Northern Ireland

Tahani Abuzeineh MB BCh CABOG
Daisy Hill Hospital, Newry, Northern Ireland

Beverley Adams MRCOG
Royal Jubilee Maternity Service, Royal Maternity Hospital, Belfast,
Northern Ireland

A member of the Hodder Headline Group
LONDON

First published in Great Britain in 2003 by
Arnold, a member of the Hodder Headline Group,
338 Euston Road, London NW1 3BH

http://www.arnoldpublishers.com

Distributed in the United States of America by
Oxford University Press Inc.,
198 Madison Avenue, New York, NY10016
Oxford is a registered trademark of Oxford University Press

Whilst the advice and information in this book are believed to be true and
accurate at the date of going to press, neither the authors nor the publisher
can accept any legal responsibility or liability for any errors or omissions
that may be made. In particular (but without limiting the generality of the
preceding disclaimer) every effort has been made to check drug dosages;
however, it is still possible that errors have been missed. Furthermore,
dosage schedules are constantly being revised and new side effects
recognized. For these reasons, the reader is strongly urged to consult the
drug companies' printed instructions before administering any of the drugs
recommended in this book.

British Library Cataloguing in Publication Data
A catalogue record for this book is available from the British Library

Library of Congress Cataloging-in-Publication Data
A catalog record for this book is available from the Library of Congress

ISBN 0 340 80927 2

1 2 3 4 5 6 7 8 9 10

Commissioning Editor: Joanna Koster
Production Editor: Wendy Rooke
Production Controller: Deborah Smith
Cover Design: Lee-May Lim

Typeset in 10/12 Minion by Phoenix Photosetting, Chatham, Kent
Printed and bound in Malta

What do you think about this book? Or any other Arnold title? Please send your comments to
feedback.arnold@hodder.co.uk

Contents

Preface

OGWW are the initials of Obstetrics and Gynaecology Wide Web. The OGWW team has been developing a vast web-based information system of protocols and guidelines for clinical practice in obstetrics and gynaecology. It is also a learning tool, and the creation of multiple choice questions was a logical next step.

This book of MCQs has been written to help you to pass the part 1 examination of the Royal College of Obstetricians and Gynaecologists. The syllabus remains broad, covering all of the basic sciences relating to the whole spectrum of obstetrics and gynaecology. Sound knowledge is essential, but candidates must also practise the technique of the exam which is equally important.

The 1200 MCQs have been designed to cover the complete syllabus with a proportionate number of questions for each topic. The structure of the questions is the same as the structure currently used in the exam; that is, a heading with five true or false stems.

The answers are detailed and are drawn from the standard texts recommended by the Royal College of Obstetricians and Gynaecologists. A complete bibliography is included at the end of the book. Some of the answers are 'augmented' with additional, relevant information (see boxed text in Answers section).

The CD-ROM you received with the book is a novel aid to learning and will help you to practise the essential technique. The questions can be selected at random to create a practice paper which you can sit under 'examination conditions'. After the mock examination, the program will calculate your score. The questions will appear in a different order every time so that you will never sit an identical exam. The answers and augmentations are the same as appear in the text.

Whether you prefer the text or the CD-ROM they will help you to prepare for the part 1 examination and, we hope, pass.

Good luck!

R de C-W,
B McE,
K El-H,
TA and BA
for the OGWW Team.

Acknowledgements

We would like to acknowledge the invaluable assistance of
Joanne McAleese, computer programmer and secretary to OGWW.

Questions

1. The following statements about vitamins are correct:
A. Vitamin K is water-soluble.
B. Vitamin D is poorly absorbed in cases of obstructive jaundice.
C. Vitamin A is a fat-soluble vitamin.
D. Vitamins supply the body with energy.
E. Vitamin D is bound to a transport protein in the circulation.

2. Vitamin B_{12}:
A. Is a fat-soluble vitamin.
B. Absorption takes place throughout the small intestine.
C. Is essential for the metabolism of folic acid in the human.
D. Deficiency leads to macrocytic anaemia.
E. Deficiency is common in strict vegetarians.

3. Folic acid:
A. Is water-soluble.
B. Requires gastric intrinsic factor for its absorption.
C. Is necessary for nucleic acid synthesis.
D. Is heat-stable.
E. Is involved in the tricarboxylic acid (Krebs) cycle.

4. Vitamin C:
A. Is found only in animal foodstuffs.
B. Is rapidly destroyed by heating.
C. There are normally large stores in the pancreas.
D. Impaired wound healing is one of the characteristic features of severe vitamin C deficiency.
E. Excess vitamin C can lead to the formation of oxalate stones in the urinary tract.

5. Vitamin B:
A. Vitamin B_1 (thiamin) deficiency leads to impaired collagen formation.
B. Vitamin B_1 (thiamin) stores in the body are adequate for up to 9 months.
C. Vitamin B_2 (riboflavin) concentration is higher in the fetus than in the mother.
D. Vitamin B_6 (pyridoxine) requirement in pregnancy is 25 mg/day.
E. Niacin is synthesized in the body from tryptophan.

6. Vitamin A (retinol):
A. Requires bile for its absorption.
B. Its deficiency leads to night blindness.
C. Its excess leads to xerophthalmia.
D. Is stored in the liver.
E. Daily dietary requirement during pregnancy is about 50 mg per day.

7. Vitamin D:
A. Is water-soluble.
B. Is stored in the body fat.
C. Is absorbed from the large intestine.
D. Deficiency leads to rickets.
E. The dietary requirement is 10 mg per day.

8. Vitamin E:
A. Is present in animal foodstuffs only.
B. Its deficiency may cause intra-uterine fetal death.
C. It potentiates the action of coumarin anticoagulants.
D. Is used in the treatment of infertility.
E. Its dietary requirement is 10 mg per day.

9. Vitamin K:
A. Is mainly found in the green leafy vegetables.
B. In adults, no external supplements are necessary.
C. Hypervitaminosis is characterized by anaemia.
D. It exists in two forms, K_1 and K_2.
E. Is stored in large quantities in the liver.

10. Regarding metabolism:
A. The metabolic rate is the amount of energy liberated per unit of time.
B. Anabolism is defined as the formation of substances which can store the energy.
C. Basal metabolic rate (BMR) is defined as the metabolic rate determined at rest in a room at 12–14 h after the last meal.
D. The BMR of a man is about 500 kcal per day.
E. The metabolic rate is decreased after consumption of a meal that is rich in protein.

11. Regarding metabolism:
A. Oxidation is the combination of a substance with either oxygen or hydrogen.
B. Co-factors are essential for certain enzyme reactions.
C. A co-enzyme is a protein substance which acts as a carrier for products of the reaction.
D. Co-enzyme A is a high-energy compound which is formed from adenine, ribose, pantothenic acid and thioethanolamine.
E. A calorie is defined as the amount of heat energy needed to raise the temperature of 1 g of water by 1 degree, from 15 to 16°C.

12. Enzymes:
A. Are proteins.
B. Heating usually results in a complete loss of enzyme activity.
C. A change in pH has no effect on the activity of an enzyme.
D. Are present in all cell organelles.
E. Organic solvents will usually destroy an enzyme's activity.

13. **Protein metabolism:**
    A. Proteins contain about 40 per cent nitrogen.
    B. Chains containing >100 amino acid residues are called proteins.
    C. Proteins yield 4 calories per gram absorbed.
    D. During pregnancy, there is a rise in the plasma concentration of triglycerides.
    E. During pregnancy, there is a rise in the plasma concentration of albumin.

14. **Uric acid:**
    A. Is the end-product of pyrimidine metabolism in humans.
    B. Is excreted mainly in the bile.
    C. Is highly soluble in body fluids.
    D. The normal blood level is 4 mg/dL.
    E. Its plasma levels do not change significantly during pregnancy.

15. **Carbohydrate metabolism:**
    A. The principal carbohydrate used in body metabolism is galactose.
    B. Glycolysis is the process of glycogen formation.
    C. The pentose shunt is active in all cells of the body except red blood cells (RBCs).
    D. The tricarboxylic acid (TCA) cycle is the common pathway for the oxidation of dietary carbohydrates, fats and proteins to CO_2 and H_2O.
    E. Acetoacetic acid and beta-hydroxybutyric acid are known as ketone bodies.

16. **Mendelian inheritance disorders:**
    A. Are caused by a defect in a single gene.
    B. The risks within an affected family are usually low and can be calculated by knowing the mode of inheritance only.
    C. Single gene defects are classified, in decreasing frequency, as dominant, recessive or X-linked.
    D. The defect may arise from a totally or partially deleted gene.
    E. If a dominant condition affects fertility, it is more likely to arise by direct inheritance.

17. **The following are examples of autosomal dominant disorders:**
    A. Achondroplasia.
    B. Acute intermittent porphyria.
    C. Alzheimer's disease.
    D. Familial hypercholesterolaemia.
    E. Tay-Sachs disease.

18. **The following are examples of X-linked disorders:**
    A. Hairy pinna.
    B. Haemophilia.
    C. Christmas disease.
    D. Multiple polyposis coli.
    E. Cystic fibrosis.

19. The following are examples of autosomal recessive disorders:
A. Sickle cell anaemia.
B. Thalassaemia major.
C. 21-Hydroxylase deficiency.
D. Galactosaemia.
E. Glycogen storage diseases.

20. Genetics:
A. Nuclear chromatin (Barr body) represents an inactivated X chromosome which must be of maternal origin.
B. An abnormal karyotype is a feature of Marfan's syndrome.
C. An abnormal karyotype is a feature of Klinefelter's syndrome.
D. An abnormal karyotype is a feature Edwards' syndrome.
E. Short stature is a phenotypic feature of Turner's syndrome.

21. Genetics:
A. Banding techniques can be used in tracing fetal autosomes to a specific parent.
B. C banding is used to distinguish between chromosomes that are similar in size and shape.
C. Chromosomes 13, 14, 15, 21 and 22 have small terminal fragments called 'satellites'.
D. Only the terminal portion of the p arm of the X chromosome remains active (Lyon hypothesis).
E. The normal Y chromosome is a submetacentric chromosome.

22. Embryology:
A. Up to weeks 6–7 of gestation, the early development of organs of reproduction is the same in both sexes.
B. The paramesonephric (Müllerian) duct degenerates and plays no functional role in the male.
C. In the male, the distal part of the mesonephric duct becomes greatly elongated and convoluted to form the epididymis.
D. In the male, the paramesonephric ducts form the vasa deferentia.
E. In the female, the paramesonephric ducts fuse to form the uterus.

23. Embryological remnants of the mesonephric tubules in the male include:
A. The utriculus masculinus.
B. The appendix of the epididymis.
C. The paradidymis.
D. The ductulus aberrans inferior.
E. The ductulus aberrans superior.

24. In the female pelvis:
A. The inlet is an oval whose longest diameter lies transversely.
B. All diameters in the mid-strait are 12 cm.
C. The transverse diameter at the level of the ischial spines is 10.5 cm.
D. The true conjugate is the antero-posterior diameter of the brim and measures about 11.5 cm.
E. The sacrum is broader than in the male.

25. **Development of the female urinary system:**
A. The ureteric bud divides repeatedly to form successive generations of collecting tubules which in turn form the major calyces, minor calyces and finally the collecting tubules of the kidney.
B. The kidneys attain their adult position during the twentieth week of fetal life.
C. Urine formation begins at about the third month of fetal life, and continues in increasing volume to term.
D. The mature fetus may well void 450 mL of urine daily into the amniotic cavity.
E. The urinary bladder is derived in part from the urogenital sinus, and in part from the ends of the mesonephric ducts.

26. **The following renal changes are typical of normal pregnancy:**
A. Increased glomerular filtration rate.
B. Increased excretion of urate.
C. Decreased excretion of folate.
D. Increased excretion of glucose.
E. Ureteric dilatation.

27. **The following physiological measurements are increased in normal healthy pregnancy:**
A. Pulse rate.
B. Cardiac output.
C. Serum colloid osmotic pressure.
D. Glomerular filtration rate.
E. PCO_2.

28. **In the normal human heart:**
A. The pressure in the pulmonary artery should not exceed 35 mmHg.
B. The pacemaker is in the sinoatrial node.
C. The Q-T interval in the electrocardiogram is the period during which ventricular depolarization and repolarization occur.
D. The pressure in the left ventricle is about 10 mmHg at the end of diastole.
E. The second heart sound has wide splitting during deep inspiration.

29. **In the normal human heart:**
A. Physical exercise increases ventricular end-diastolic volume.
B. Stimulation of the sympathetic nerve supply to the heart affects ventricular end-diastolic volume.
C. Myocardial contractility is reduced in acidosis.
D. During normal pregnancy there is an increase in the arteriovenous oxygen gradient.
E. Myocardial contractility is reduced in treatment with ritodrine.

30. Regarding the respiratory system:
A. Alveolar air in the lungs is fully saturated with water.
B. In a healthy resting individual, the total respiratory dead space volume has almost equal anatomical and alveolar components.
C. The functional residual capacity is reduced during normal pregnancy.
D. During pregnancy there is an increase in the respiratory rate.
E. Intrapleural pressure may exceed atmospheric pressure at the end of forced expiration.

31. In the neonate:
A. The bowel is sterile at birth.
B. The respiratory rate is in the region of 25–35 per minute.
C. The ductus arteriosus closes functionally within an hour of birth.
D. Compared with the adult, the neonate has higher blood levels of vitamin K.
E. Compared with the adult, the neonate has reduced blood levels of clotting factor X.

32. During pregnancy there an increase in:
A. Fibrinolytic activity.
B. Antithrombin III concentration.
C. The total lung capacity.
D. Plasma osmolality.
E. The proportion of B to T lymphocytes.

33. The small intestine:
A. In life is about 3 m (9 ft) long.
B. Paneth cells have no known function.
C. Villi are shorter in the jejunum than in the ileum.
D. Circular folds (valves of Kerckring) are more frequent in the ileum than in the jejunum.
E. Lining cells (enterocytes) have the fastest turnover rate of any cells in the body.

34. Gastrin:
A. Its fasting plasma concentrations are abnormally high in most patients after vagotomy for duodenal ulcer.
B. Vasoactive intestinal polypeptide (VIP) inhibits its secretion.
C. Protein in the duodenum inhibits its secretion.
D. Stimulates secretion of pepsinogen more strongly than secretion of hydrogen ions.
E. Is elaborated in 'G-cells' that are confined to the antral region of the stomach.

35. Fetal blood:
A. During the 6th week of embryonic life, extramedullary haematopoiesis begins mainly in the liver and spleen.
B. Most haemoglobin in the fetus is HbF chains, in place of the adult haemoglobins HbA and HbA_2.
C. Fetal red blood cells are smaller than maternal blood cells.
D. Fetal red blood cells are more resistant than adult cells to osmotic lysis by alkali and/or acid.
E. At birth, the mean capillary haemoglobin level is 12 g/dL.

36. White blood cells:
A. Basophilic granules contain histamine and heparin.
B. Eosinophils attack parasites and produce leukotrienes.
C. The half-life of neutrophils is 14 days.
D. The half-life of monocytes in tissue is 72 h.
E. After birth, most of the lymphocytes are formed in the bone marrow.

37. In the fetus:
A. Urine production is increased with advanced gestation.
B. Fetal haemoglobin has a high affinity for oxygen.
C. Lung surfactants contain up to 8 per cent proteins.
D. Glycogen storage in the liver increases towards term.
E. Fetal breathing movements increase within 72 h of the onset of labour.

38. The following statements are true about normally distributed data:
A. The mean and mode will be equal.
B. Some 97.5% of the observations will be within 2 standard deviations (SDs) of the mean.
C. Student's t-test can be used to test the difference between two means.
D. Non-parametric tests cannot be used to compare sets of data.
E. When analysing the results of a 2×2 table there will be one degree of freedom.

39. Red blood cells (RBCs):
A. The half-life is 6 weeks.
B. Carry haemoglobin.
C. Are biconcave disks.
D. Have a nucleus.
E. An adult human has 200 g of haemoglobin in the circulating blood.

40. Streptococci:
A. Are penicillin-resistant bacteria.
B. Are oval in shape.
C. Are arranged in chains.
D. Produce endotoxin.
E. Produce hyaluronidase.

41. Beta-haemolytic streptococci:
A. Cause localized infections.
B. Are classified according to Lancefield groups, based on cell-wall carbohydrate antigen.
C. Group A haemolytic streptococci are found in the throat in 25 per cent of normal adults and children.
D. They cause sore throat and erysipilis.
E. Group A haemolytic streptococcus is the most common pathogenic organism.

42. *Staphylococcus aureus*:
A. Is arranged in chains.
B. Is non-motile.
C. Is a facultative anaerobe.
D. Is a spore-forming bacterium.
E. Is a penicillin-resistant bacterium.

43. *Staphylococcus aureus*:
A. Produces a golden-yellow colony pigmentation.
B. Is mostly pathogenic.
C. Produces coagulase.
D. Produces exotoxin (enterotoxin).
E. Is non-haemolytic.

44. *Listeria monocytogenes*:
A. Is a non-motile bacterium.
B. Is a Gram-positive coccus.
C. Can be found in soft cheese and milk.
D. Produces haemolysins.
E. Resists freezing.

45. *Listeria monocytogenes*:
A. Can be diagnosed by blood culture.
B. Is sensitive to alkaline conditions.
C. Has an ability to grow in salt.
D. Infection is treated with ampicillin.
E. Can lead to miscarriage.

46. Gonococcus:
A. Is a Gram-positive diplococcus bacillus.
B. Is treated with penicillin.
C. Can penetrate the stratified squamous epithelium.
D. Is sensitive to cold.
E. In the male it may cause an acute suppurative urethritis and proctitis.

47. The following are Gram-positive bacilli:
A. Anthrax.
B. *Mycobacterium.*
C. *Lactobacillus.*
D. *Clostridium.*
E. *Salmonella.*

48. The following statements are true:
A. Döderlein's bacillus is Gram-positive.
B. *Corynebacterium diphtheriae* produces exotoxin.
C. *Corynebacterium diphtheriae* is Gram-negative.
D. Döderlein's bacillus is predominant in the vagina at birth.
E. Schick's test is a diagnostic test for diphtheria.

49. Clostridia
A. *Clostridium tetani* produces a neurotoxin.
B. *Clostridium welchii* gives a positive Neglar reaction.
C. *Clostridium welchii* causes gas gangrene.
D. *Clostridium botulinum* can lead to food poisoning.
E. *Clostridium tetani* have drumstick spores (terminal).

50. *Bacteroides* is:
A. Anaerobic.
B. Gram-positive.
C. Non-spore-forming.
D. Sensitive to metronidazole.
E. A cause of bacterial vaginosis.

51. Food poisoning can be caused by:
A. *Clostridium welchii.*
B. Streptococci.
C. *Campylobacter.*
D. *Clostridium botulinum.*
E. *Bacillus cereus.*

52. *Mycobacterium tuberculosis*:
A. Is motile.
B. Is anaerobic.
C. Is very sensitive to drying.
D. Is acid- and alcohol-fast.
E. Is easy to culture.

53. *Treponema pallidum* (syphilis):
A. Only affects humans.
B. Its incubation period is 2–3 weeks.
C. May only be visualized by dark-ground illumination.
D. Is sensitive to water and drying.
E. Crosses the placenta before 12 weeks' gestation.

54. *Chlamydia*:
A. Is motile.
B. Is Gram-positive.
C. Is the most common sexually transmitted disease.
D. Causes Fitz-Hugh–Curtis syndrome.
E. Causes lymphogranuloma venereum.

55. Which of the following pairs of infections and complications are correct?
A. Deafness: *Toxoplasma gondii*.
B. Cardiac anomalies: Coxsackie B virus.
C. Hydrocephalus: *Toxoplasma gondii*.
D. Cataracts: *Rubella*.
E. Encephalitis: herpes simplex type I.

56. The following are DNA-containing viruses:
A. Varicella zoster.
B. Smallpox.
C. Papillomavirus.
D. Hepatitis B.
E. Mumps.

57. AIDS:
A. Is caused by an RNA virus.
B. Its incubation period is 12 months.
C. An incomplete virus will not have the same effect.
D. Is associated with Kaposi's sarcoma.
E. The causative virus binds to the CD4 molecule on T cells.

58. In statistics:
A. The standard deviation is the square-root of the variance.
B. Non-parametric tests cannot be used in normally distributed data.
C. The incidence of a disorder is the rate of occurrence of new cases in a defined population in a period of time.
D. In any set of observations the mean is always less than the mode.
E. In an even set of numbers the median value is the average of the middle two numbers.

59. In statistics:
A. The mode of a distribution is the least frequently occurring value.
B. Wilcoxon's rank sum test is a non-parametric test.
C. In any set of observations half of the observations are greater than the median.
D. The chi-square test compares the observed and expected frequencies of an event.
E. Infant mortality rate is the number of infants dying during the first year per 10 000 live births.

60. **In diagnostic ultrasound:**
A. Ultrasound is generated by the effect of electricity on a ceramic crystal.
B. Resolution increases with increased frequency.
C. Medical ultrasound uses the range of 1000–5000 kilohertz (kHz).
D. Attenuation increases with increased frequency.
E. Ultrasound velocity in any given medium is constant.

61. **Glomerular filtration rate may be measured using:**
A. Insulin.
B. Para-aminohippuric acid.
C. Glucagon.
D. Glucose.
E. Inulin.

62. **During pregnancy there is an increase in the following:**
A. Total white cell count.
B. Lymphocytes.
C. Erythrocyte sedimentation rate.
D. Alkaline phosphatase.
E. Haemoglobin concentration.

63. **In pregnancy:**
A. Fetal growth is affected by maternal diet.
B. Maternal weight gain is maximum during mid-pregnancy.
C. Meconium is not present before 24 weeks' gestation.
D. Osteoclastic activity is increased.
E. Gallbladder motility is increased.

64. **In acid–base balance:**
A. The normal pH of arterial blood is 7.4.
B. Magnesium bicarbonate is a buffer.
C. The placenta is permeable to hydrogen ions.
D. In metabolic acidosis, there is an excess of fixed acids.
E. Respiratory acidosis is associated with decreased level of CO_2.

65. **Normal urodynamic findings in the adult female:**
A. Voiding pressure: 45–70 mmHg.
B. Residual urine: 50 mL.
C. First sensation of bladder filling: 150–200 mL.
D. Maximum voiding pressure: 70 cm H_2O.
E. Bladder capacity: 400–600 mL.

66. Serological tests are used to:

A. Diagnose infections.
B. Identify micro-organisms.
C. Type blood for blood banks.
D. Type tissues for transplantaion.
E. Study antigen–antibody interaction.

67. The following are true about serological tests:

A. Between 2 and 4 weeks must elapse before IgG antibodies produced in response to infection are detectable.
B. In the laboratory diagnosis of viral infection a single sample is collected during the acute phase and stored at $-20°C$ prior to analysis.
C. The Elek test is used to detect diphtheria toxin from isolates of *Corynebacterium diphtheriae*.
D. Haemagglutination inhibition is used to detect the presence of antibodies to influenza virus in a patient's serum.
E. The Paul–Bunnell test is used to detect infectious mononucleosis.

68. Sexually transmitted diseases (STDs):

A. The incidence of most STDs is decreasing.
B. Papillomaviruses are the most common of all STDs.
C. Syphilis is caused by the spirochete *Treponema pallidum*.
D. The VDRL test (Venereal Disease Reference Laboratory) is a non-specific test for syphilis.
E. Gonorrhoea is caused by a Gram-positive organism.

69. A vaccine should be:

A. Effective.
B. Safe.
C. Stable.
D. Inexpensive.
E. Easy to administer.

70. The effectiveness of a vaccine:

A. Is purely due to antibody response in tuberculosis.
B. Is a purely cell-mediated response in streptococcal pneumonia.
C. Is due to high levels of serum antibody in mucosal protection against polio.
D. Is due to activation of cytotoxic cells in hepatitis.
E. Can be measured by checking circulating IgG titres in rubella.

71. Regarding attenuated vaccines:

A. The virulence has been artificially reduced.
B. Adaptation to high temperatures is one of the two methods used to produce live attenuated vaccines.
C. Make up the bulk of successful viral vaccines.
D. The killed (inactivated) form of the polio vaccine is known as the Salker vaccine.
E. Rubella vaccine is not a 'live' attenuated vaccine.

72. Killed or 'inactivated' organisms include:
A. Influenza.
B. Hepatitis A.
C. *Salmonella typhi.*
D. Measles.
E. Mumps.

73. Pathological consequences of the immune response:
A. The most widely used classification of hypersensitivity is that of Coombs and Gell.
B. Type 1 hypersensitivity is a cytotoxic reaction.
C. Part of the mechanism involved in mediating type 3 hypersensitivity is also involved in protective immunity.
D. The main effectors of cell-mediated immunity are T cells.
E. Rejection of allografts is an expression of cell-mediated immunity.

74. The following are examples of type 4 (cell-mediated) hypersensitivity:
A. Tuberculosis.
B. Schistosomiasis (eggs).
C. Actinomycosis.
D. Mycoplasma.
E. African trypanosomiasis.

75. The menopause:
A. The length of the menstrual cycle increases, beginning 2 to 8 years before the menopause.
B. The duration of the luteal phase is the major determinant of cycle length.
C. Menstrual cycle changes prior to the menopause are marked by elevated follicle-stimulating hormone (FSH) and inhibin.
D. Eventually there is a 10- to 20-fold increase in mean serum levels of FSH.
E. Luteinizing hormone (LH) levels are higher than FSH because FSH is cleared from the blood so much faster.

76. The menopause:
A. The postmenopausal ovary in most women secretes more testosterone than the premenopausal ovary.
B. The circulating oestradiol level after menopause is approximately 10–20 pg/mL (40–70 pmol/L).
C. 'Hot flushes' are more frequent and severe during the day.
D. The flush persists for longer than 5 years in as many as 25–50 per cent of women.
E. The flush coincides with a surge in follicle-stimulating hormone (FSH).

77. After the menopause:

A. Oestrogen therapy increases the rapid eye movement (REM) sleep time.
B. Trabecular bone resorption and formation occurs four to eight times as fast as cortical bone.
C. Cortical bone is responsible for 80 per cent of total bone.
D. Five per cent of total bone mass loss will occur per year after the menopause.
E. The critical blood level of oestradiol that is necessary to maintain bone is 40–50 pg/mL (150–180 pmol/L).

78. Human chorionic gonadotrophin (hCG):

A. Is a glycoprotein with a half-life of 2 h.
B. Consists of two covalently linked subunits called alpha (a) and beta (b).
C. The a-subunit is common to hCG, follicle-stimulating hormone (FSH), luteinizing hormone (LH) and thyroid-stimulating hormone (TSH).
D. HCG is secreted by the syncytiotrophoblast.
E. HCG can be detected in the blood of normal men.

79. Human chorionic gonadotrophin (hCG) levels in maternal serum:

A. The maternal circulating hCG concentration is approximately 100 IU/L at the time of the expected but missed menses.
B. A maximal hCG level of 100 000 IU/L is reached at 18–20 weeks' gestation.
C. After peaking, hCG levels decrease steadily until term.
D. hCG levels close to term are higher in women bearing female fetuses.
E. When the titre exceeds 1000–1500 IU/L, vaginal ultrasonography should identify the presence of an intra-uterine gestational sac.

80. Human placental lactogen (hPL):

A. Is a single-chain polypeptide of 191 amino acids held together by two disulphide bonds.
B. Has a long half-life of 48 h.
C. Is very similar in structure to human growth hormone (hGH) and has over 90 per cent of hGH somatotrophin activity.
D. The growth hormone hPL gene family consists of five genes on chromosome 17.
E. Blood levels of hPL are decreased in the presence of hypoglycaemia.

81. Human placental lactogen (hPL):

A. The level in the maternal circulation is correlated with fetal and placental weight.
B. Its metabolic role is to mobilize lipids as free fatty acids.
C. Induces insulin resistance and carbohydrate intolerance.
D. When glucose becomes scarce for the fetus, hPL increases the transport of fatty acids across the placenta.
E. Fetal undernutrition can lead to insulin resistance in later life.

82. Angiotensin-converting enzyme inhibitors:
A. Impair fetal renal function.
B. Are associated with polyhydramnios.
C. May cause fetal death in later pregnancy.
D. Should be stopped before conception.
E. Can be safely used in the puerperium.

83. Alpha-methyldopa:
A. Is the most tested antihypertensive drug for use in pregnancy.
B. The dose range is 1–3 mg daily.
C. Is relatively contra-indicated in the puerperium.
D. Adverse effects include insomnia and agitation.
E. Calcium-channel blockers are useful to augment the action of methyldopa.

84. Beta-adrenoceptor blocking drugs:
A. May exacerbate asthma.
B. Cause intra-uterine growth retardation when given from early pregnancy.
C. Labetalol is a pure beta-blocker, and is the oral agent of choice in the UK for treating severe pre-eclamptic hypertension.
D. Labetalol has intrinsic sympathomimetic activity (ISA).
E. Are contra-indicated in diabetes mellitus.

85. Drugs and breast-feeding:
A. Ranitidine is safe to use as it is not secreted in breast milk.
B. Methyldopa is the drug of choice to treat hypertension during the puerperium.
C. Angiotensin-converting enzyme (ACE) inhibitors may be used safely during the puerperium.
D. Thiazide diuretics have been shown to increase milk production.
E. The combination of co-amoxiclav (Augmentin) and metronidazole (Flagyl) is recommended to treat puerperal infection in breast-feeding mothers.

86. Systemic lupus erythematosus (SLE) and pregnancy:
A. In women, SLE has a prevalence of about 1 in 1000.
B. In women with glomerulonephritis and a serum creatinine concentration >130 mmol/L before conception, only 10 per cent of the babies will be born alive.
C. The optimal situation is control of disease activity for at least 6 months before conception, without the use of cytotoxic agents.
D. Pre-eclampsia is difficult to distinguish from worsening lupus nephritis.
E. Patients with SLE renal involvement are advised to take aspirin 75 mg daily throughout pregnancy.

87. Systemic lupus erythematosus (SLE) and the neonate:
A. Neonatal SLE usually results from passively acquired maternal anti-Ro antigens.
B. The most common fetal condition is congenital heart block.
C. Congenital heart block occurs due to maternal autoantibodies causing reversible damage to the fetal cardiac conducting system.
D. Two-thirds of surviving neonates with heart block will require a pacemaker.
E. High-dose corticosteroids significantly improve fetal outcome.

88. Rheumatoid arthritis (RA):
A. Pregnancy alleviates the symptoms of RA.
B. Exacerbations of RA tend to occur in the puerperium.
C. RA does not adversely affect pregnancy.
D. Treatment of RA with azathioprine during pregnancy may weaken fetal collagen.
E. Methotrexate may be used for symptom control of RA in pregnancy.

89. The antiphospholipid syndrome:
A. Some healthy individuals have antiphospholipid antibodies without symptoms.
B. Fewer than 20 per cent of babies are born alive to mothers with untreated antiphospholipid syndrome.
C. Is characterized by high levels of anticardiolipin antibodies.
D. In labour, patients who regularly took 7.5 mg or more of prednisolone per day during the fortnight before delivery should continue on this dose.
E. Patients who are taking non-steroidal anti-inflammatory drugs (NSAIDs) are recommended not to breast-feed.

90. The pancreas:
A. Is made up of two types of tissue, fibrous stroma and islets of Langerhans.
B. The islets of Langerhans are made up of two types of cells: a (alpha) cells; and b (beta) cells.
C. Alpha cells produce glucagons.
D. Delta (d) cells produce insulin.
E. The glandular acini are responsible for the secretion of bicarbonate and enzymes.

91. In the female pelvis:
A. All diameters are smaller than in the male.
B. The sub-pubic arch is about 80–85 degrees.
C. The sacral promontory is more prominent.
D. The obturator foramen is triangular.
E. The sacrum is broader in the male.

92. Insulin:
A. Is a polypeptide molecule, with a molecular weight of 5734 daltons.
B. Consists of 51 amino acids.
C. The amino acid residues form two chains, A and B, which are joined by two covalent bonds.
D. Zinc is needed for the crystallization of insulin.
E. The pancreas stores about 2500 units of insulin at any one time.

93. Insulin:
A. The fasting plasma level of insulin is about 10 mU/mL.
B. The half-life of insulin is 2 h.
C. Insulin is degraded in the liver and kidneys by the enzyme glutathione insulin transhydrogenase.
D. Human sequence insulin may be produced biosynthetically by recombinant DNA technology using *E. coli*.
E. Is effective orally if given in higher doses.

94. Insulin release is stimulated by:
A. Adrenaline.
B. Noradrenaline.
C. Glucose.
D. Amino acids.
E. Free fatty acids.

95. Glucagon:
A. Is a polypeptide consisting of 129 amino acids.
B. Is secreted by the alpha cells of the islets of Langerhans.
C. The release of glucagon results in the rapid mobilization of hepatic glucose by gluconeogenesis.
D. Is used to treat hypoglycaemic reactions in insulin-dependent diabetics.
E. Is contra-indicated in phaeochromocytoma.

96. Glucagon release is stimulated by:
A. Hypoglycaemia.
B. Exercise.
C. Adrenaline.
D. Free fatty acids.
E. Insulin.

97. The femoral triangle:
A. Is a triangular area situated in the upper part of the lateral aspect of the thigh.
B. Is bounded superiorly by the inguinal ligament.
C. Is bounded medially by the sartorius muscle.
D. Is bounded medially by the medial borders of the adductor longus muscle.
E. The muscles lying in the floor of the femoral triangle are iliacus, psoas major, pectineus, part of adductor brevis and adductor magnus.

98. The femoral triangle:
A. The floor is gutter-shaped and formed from lateral to medial by the iliopsoas, the pectineus and the adductor longus.
B. The roof is formed by the skin and fascia of the thigh.
C. Contains the terminal part of the femoral nerve and its branches, the femoral sheath, the femoral artery and its branches, the femoral vein and its tributaries and the deep inguinal lymph nodes.
D. The base of the triangle is formed by the inguinal ligament, the lateral border by the sartorius muscle and the medial border by the adductor longus muscle.
E. In the femoral triangle the femoral artery lies on the psoas muscle.

99. Regarding the pelvic skeleton:
A. It is made up by the innominate bone, the sacrum and the fifth lumbar vertebra.
B. The sacrum has five sacral foramina.
C. The obturator foramen transmits the obturator nerve and vessels.
D. The innominate bone consists of the ilium and pubis.
E. The greater sciatic foramen transmits the piriformis muscle, the superior and inferior gluteal vessels and nerve.

100. The ischio-rectal fossa(e):
A. Is a wedge-shaped space on each side of the anal canal.
B. Is filled with dense fat.
C. Lies lateral to the pudendal canal.
D. Are separated from each other by the vagina.
E. The lateral wall is formed by the obturator internus muscle covered with pelvic fascia.

101. In the anterior abdominal wall:
A. The external oblique arises from the lower five ribs.
B. The inguinal canal contains the round ligament.
C. The nerve supply is from T6 to T12 and L1.
D. The pyramidalis muscle is always absent.
E. The superior epigastric artery lies superficial to the rectus abdominis.

102. The vulva:
A. The urethral fold fuses, as in the male, to develop into labia minora.
B. The nerve endings of the vestibule are mostly free, with few or no corpuscles.
C. The blood supply of the labia majora is exclusively derived from internal pudendal artery.
D. The labia majora contain Ruffini corpuscles.
E. The Bartholin's gland is normally not palpable.

103. The vagina:
A. The paramesonephric duct gives rise to both the uterus and the entire vagina.
B. Is 7–10 cm long.
C. The urogenital sinus gives rise to part of the vagina and the proximal part of the urethra.
D. Becomes canalized at 22 weeks of gestational age.
E. Vaginal fluid has a lower potassium concentration than plasma.

104. In the vagina:
A. A double vagina or atresia of the vagina results from premature fusion of sinovaginal bulbs.
B. The pH is 4–5 during child-bearing years.
C. The upper vagina is sensitive only to stretch.
D. The lymphatics of the lower part of vagina drain to the sacral nodes.
E. The blood supply of the vagina is mainly from the uterine artery.

105. The uterus:
A. The upper portions of the Müllerian ducts fuse to form the uterus.
B. The uterus is supported only by the levator ani muscles.
C. The peritoneum covers the entire uterus posteriorly.
D. The increased blood supply to the uterus in normal pregnancy is attributed to increased levels of angiotensin II.
E. The uterus fails to acquire an anteverted position in 5 per cent of women.

106. Oxytocin:
A. Is a nonapeptide.
B. Is released by the fetus during labour.
C. Is released in the male during orgasm.
D. Causes milk ejection.
E. Is inactivated by oxytocinase.

107. The uterus:
A. There is no submucosa in the uterus.
B. The blood supply of the uterus is entirely from the uterine artery.
C. The lymphatic drainage of the fundus of the uterus is into the para-aortic nodes.
D. The broad ligament has no supporting function to the uterus.
E. The nerves of the uterus are branches of the superior hypogastric plexus.

108. The cervix:
A. The external os of the cervix is normally on a level with the ischial spines.
B. The posterior surface of the cervix is partially covered by peritoneum.
C. Cervical mucus becomes profuse and clear under the action of oestrogen before ovulation.
D. The endocervical canal is lined by transitional epithelium.
E. Is largely composed of fibrous tissue.

109. The uterus and cervix:
A. The body of the uterus and cervix are relatively insensitive to cutting and burning.
B. The cavity of the uterus, as in the cervix, is fusiform in shape.
C. The endometrial and cervical lining are shed at menstruation.
D. The lymphatics of the cervix drain to the external and internal iliac nodes.
E. In pregnancy the internal os is located in the cervix rather than the isthmus.

110. The right ovary:
A. Is covered by peritoneum in the adult.
B. Receives its blood supply from the internal iliac artery.
C. Has the ovarian ligament attached to its medial pole.
D. Its venous drainage is to the right renal vein.
E. Has lymphatic drainage to the internal iliac nodes.

111. The ovary:
A. The normal ovary measures 4×2 cm.
B. In postmenopausal women, the ovaries become smaller and shrunken and are covered in scar tissue.
C. The round ligament of the ovary and the round ligament of the uterus constitute the gubernaculum.
D. The ovaries originate from the same embryogenic structure as the suprarenal glands.
E. The obturator artery crosses the floor of the ovarian fossa.

112. The ovary:
A. The ovaries do not descend into the pelvic cavity until childhood.
B. The ovarian artery arises from the aorta at the level of the third lumbar vertebra.
C. The ureter passes in front of the ovary at the level of the bifurcation of the iliac arteries.
D. The nerve supply to the ovary is derived exclusively from parasympathetic fibres.
E. During pregnancy the enlarged uterus pushes the ovaries down into the pelvis.

113. The ureter:
A. The early splitting of the ureteric bud may result in partial or complete duplication of the ureter.
B. The muscular layer of the ureter consists of longitudinal and circular layers throughout its whole length.
C. Is crossed by the genitofemoral nerve.
D. Has a squamous epithelium.
E. Is more dilated on the right side in pregnancy.

114. The ureter:
A. Is 10–15 cm in length.
B. Is of endodermal origin.
C. Its blood supply is mainly from the aorta.
D. The ureter runs above the lateral fornix of the vagina, 2 cm lateral to the cervix.
E. The ureter is crossed superficially by the gonadal vessels.

115. The internal iliac artery:
A. Divides into anterior and posterior divisions at the upper border of the lesser sciatic foramen.
B. The median sacral artery arises from the posterior division.
C. At the level of the sacroiliac joint it is crossed anteriorly by the ureter.
D. The superior gluteal artery arises from the anterior division.
E. The superior and inferior vesical arteries arise from the umbilical artery.

116. **The lumbar plexus:**
A. The ilioinguinal nerve arises from the anterior primary ramus of L1.
B. Lies posterior to the piriformis muscle.
C. The obturator and the femoral nerves arise from anterior divisions of L2–L4.
D. The iliohypogastric nerve arises from L1.
E. The obturator nerve supplies the obturator internus, adductor longus and adductor brevis muscles.

117. **Regarding the sacral plexus and its branches:**
A. The plexus lies in front of piriformis muscle and behind the ureter.
B. The perforating cutaneous nerve arises from S2, S3.
C. The accessory obturator nerve arises from S3, S4.
D. The sciatic nerve divides into the common peroneal and tibial nerves above the popliteal fossa.
E. The first sacral root contributes to the anterior tibial nerve.

118. **The inguinal canal:**
A. The inguinal ligament is situated in front of iliacus muscle and the femoral nerve.
B. The posterior wall of the canal is formed along its entire length by the fascia transversalis.
C. The superficial inguinal ring is a triangle-shaped defect in the aponeurosis of the internal oblique muscle.
D. The ilioinguinal nerve lies above the inguinal ligament.
E. In the female, the only structures that pass through the inguinal canal from the abdominal cavity are the round ligament and a few lymph vessels.

119. **The aorta:**
A. Enters the abdomen at the level of the twelfth thoracic vertebra.
B. It divides into the two common iliac arteries in front of the fifth lumbar vertebra.
C. The common iliac arteries divide into external and internal iliac arteries in front of the sacroiliac joint.
D. The external iliac artery runs along the lateral border of the psoas major muscle.
E. The superior mesenteric artery is a posterior visceral branch of the aorta.

120. **Uterine vessels:**
A. The uterine artery arises from the anterior division of internal iliac artery.
B. The uterine artery crosses above the ureter and reaches the cervix at the level of the internal os.
C. The uterine artery, along with the vaginal and ovarian arteries, enlarges during pregnancy.
D. The uterine veins do not have surrounding supporting sheaths.
E. The uterine vein drains into the external iliac vein.

121. Regarding the branches of the aorta:
A. The coeliac artery supplies the gastro-intestinal tract from the middle of the second part of the duodenum as far as the distal one-third of the transverse colon.
B. The coeliac trunk arises from the aorta between the right and the left crura of the diaphragm.
C. The superior mesenteric artery arises from the aorta at the level of the first lumbar vertebra.
D. The left colic artery is the larger terminal branch of the superior mesenteric artery.
E. The inferior mesenteric artery arises from the front of the aorta at the upper border of the third part of the duodenum at the level of the umbilicus.

122. Regarding the inguinal canal:
A. It is 10 cm (4 inches) long in the adult.
B. The deep inguinal ring is an oval opening in the fascia transversalis.
C. Its floor is formed by the grooved surface of the inguinal ligament and at its lateral end by the lacunar ligament.
D. The inguinal ligament extends from the anterior inferior iliac spine to the pubic tubercle.
E. The inferior epigastric artery runs medial to the deep inguinal ring.

123. The pudendal nerve:
A. Leaves the main pelvic cavity through the greater sciatic foramen.
B. The inferior rectal nerve (which is a branch of the pudendal nerve) supplies the internal anal sphincter.
C. Arises from S2–S3 nerve roots.
D. The pudendal nerve and internal pudendal vessels are embedded in a fascial canal (pudendal canal) in the medial wall of the ischiorectal fossa.
E. The superior haemorrhoidal nerve is one of its terminal branches.

124. Nerves:
A. The phrenic nerve arises from the posterior rami of C3–C5.
B. The femoral nerve supplies psoas major and iliacus.
C. The phrenic nerve has a contribution to the suprarenal glands.
D. The levator ani muscle is innervated by S2–S4.
E. The obturator nerve provides articulate branches to the hip and knee joints.

125. The ischio-rectal fossa:
A. The two fossae do not communicate with each other.
B. Contains the perineal nerve in its posterior part.
C. Lies inferior to the levator ani.
D. The anal canal and the sloping levator ani muscles form the medial wall of each fossa.
E. Contains the middle rectal artery.

126. Regarding the pituitary gland:
A. It is entirely mesodermal in origin.
B. It is situated in the posterior cranial fossa.
C. The hypothalamus lies above the pituitary gland.
D. It has a portal circulation.
E. Vasopressin is secreted by the posterior lobe.

127. The fetal ovary:
A. The ovarian ligament is a derivative of the mesonephric fold.
B. The ligament of the ovary is the homologue of the gubernaculum of the testis in the male.
C. The number of oocytes is greatest during fetal life, and declines thereafter.
D. In early fetal life the ovaries lie in the hypochondrial region.
E. Is covered by peritoneum.

128. Prolactin:
A. Is structurally related to human placental lactogen (hPL).
B. Its secretion is stimulated by dopamine.
C. Has a molecular weight of 100 000 daltons.
D. Its release is pulsatile.
E. Is produced by the basophil cells of the anterior lobe of the pituitary gland.

129. Growth hormone (GH):
A. Is a glycoprotein hormone.
B. Secretion is markedly increased during pregnancy.
C. Is responsible for growth in children and in the fetus.
D. Secretion is increased by hypoglycaemia.
E. Pygmies have low levels of GH.

130. Adrenocorticotrophic hormone (ACTH):
A. Is a polypeptide hormone.
B. Has a molecular weight of 4500 daltons.
C. Is the main hormone controlling aldosterone secretion.
D. Secretion is increased in congenital adrenal hyperplasia.
E. Contains the sequence of alpha-melanocyte-stimulating hormone.

131. The anterior pituitary:
A. Lies above the optic chiasma.
B. Produces oxytocin.
C. Has basophil cells which secrete luteinizing hormone (LH).
D. Develops from the alimentary tract.
E. Has a direct neuroregulatory mechanism.

132. Prolactin:
A. Release is stimulated by thyrotrophin-releasing hormone (TRH).
B. Secretion is inhibited by sexual intercourse.
C. Is a protein hormone.
D. Concentration in the plasma rises in human pregnancy.
E. Has a half-life of 6 hours.

133. Oxytocin:
A. Is secreted by the posterior pituitary.
B. Alcohol stimulates the release of oxytocin.
C. Is composed of 50 amino acids.
D. Is relatively inactive in early pregnancy.
E. Has some antidiuretic action.

134. The anterior pituitary:
A. Lies in the sella turcica.
B. Lies below the hypothalamus.
C. Produces oestradiol.
D. Increases in weight during pregnancy.
E. Acidophils secrete prolactin and growth hormone.

135. The hypothalamus:
A. Stretches from the optic chiasma in front to the mamillary bodies behind.
B. Forms part of the mid-brain.
C. Is responsible for temperature regulation.
D. Has nerve connections with the anterior lobe of the pituitary gland.
E. Forms part of the roof of the third ventricle.

136. The hypothalamus:
A. Secretes releasing hormones which are concerned in the control of mammary gland secretion.
B. The principal afferent and efferent neural pathways to and from the hypothalamus are unmyelinated.
C. The portal hypophyseal vessels form a direct vascular link between the hypothalamus and the posterior pituitary.
D. The hypothalamus regulates body temperature through its connection with the limbic system.
E. The median eminence is outside the blood–brain barrier.

137. Vasopressin:
A. Is a nonapeptide hormone.
B. Secretion is inhibited by alcohol.
C. May elevate arterial blood pressure by direct action on the arteriolar smooth muscles.
D. Secretion is increased by angiotensin II.
E. Is produced in excess in diabetes insipidus.

138. The posterior pituitary:
A. Is a neurosecretory gland.
B. Secretes gonadotrophin-releasing hormone (GnRH).
C. Releases hormones which affect the growth of the placenta.
D. Produces vasopressin, which increases the permeability of the collecting ducts of the kidney to water.
E. Is neuroectodermal in origin.

139. Releasing hormones:
A. Releasing hormones are polypeptides.
B. The greater the secretion of endogenous releasing hormone, the lesser is the response to exogenous releasing factors.
C. Gonadotrophin-releasing hormone (GnRH) is released as a series of pulses into the portal vessels.
D. Corticotrophin-releasing hormone (CRH) is composed of 14 amino acids.
E. Vasoactive polypeptide (VIP) is a potent releaser of prolactin.

140. Follicle-stimulating hormone (FSH):
A. FSH is a glycoprotein composed of two subunits, alpha and gamma.
B. The alpha chain is composed of 92 amino acids.
C. The receptors for FSH are serpentine receptors coupled to adenyl cyclase.
D. Is produced by the posterior pituitary gland.
E. It is responsible for the final maturation of the ovarian follicles, and oestrogen secretion from them.

141. Follicle-stimulating hormone (FSH):
A. The half-life of human FSH is the same as luteinizing hormone (LH): about 170 min.
B. The molecular weight of FSH is 28 000 daltons.
C. In the male, FSH is concerned with maintenance and growth of the germinal epithelium of the seminiferous tubules and with sperm production.
D. Gonadotrophin-releasing hormone (GnRH), released in less frequent pulses, causes no change in FSH secretion.
E. Is excreted in small amounts at the climacteric.

142. Luteinizing hormone (LH):
A. LH is responsible for ovulation and the initial formation of the corpus luteum.
B. The molecular weight of LH is 28 000 daltons.
C. Sustained continuous administration of exogenous gonadotrophin-releasing hormone (GnRH) analogues leads to increased production of LH.
D. LH has highest pulse frequency during the late follicular phase.
E. The highest pulse amplitude is during the late luteal phase.

143. Luteinizing hormone (LH):

A. The circulating half-life is mainly proportional to the amount of sialic acid present.
B. Is secreted from the anterior pituitary gland.
C. The beta chain is similar to that of follicle-stimulating hormone (FSH) and thyroid-stimulating hormone (TSH).
D. In the male, LH maintains the interstitial cells of the testes and stimulates them to secrete testosterone.
E. An LH surge occurs 36 h prior to ovulation.

144. Steroid hormones:

A. Hyperthyroidism increases sex hormone-binding globulin (SHBG) levels.
B. The majority of the principal sex steroids are bound to albumin.
C. The first step of steroid hormone formation from cholesterol occurs in the endoplasmic reticulum.
D. Adrenocorticotrophic hormone (ACTH) stimulates the conversion of cholesterol to pregnenolone, and also later biosynthetic steps.
E. Corticosteroids are degraded and conjugated with glucuronic acid in the liver, but are excreted by the kidneys.

145. Ovulation:

A. Regular menstruation indicates regular ovulation.
B. The LH surge stimulates continuation of reduction division in the oocyte, luteinization of the granulosa and synthesis of progesterone and prostaglandins within the follicle.
C. Ovulation appears to alternate between the two ovaries.
D. Premenstrual mastalgia is reliable clinical evidence that ovulation has occurred.
E. In lactating women, ovulation is most unlikely up to 6 months.

146. Ovulation:

A. Ovulation occurs during the hours after the oestrogen peak.
B. Progesterone enhances the activity of proteolytic enzymes responsible, together with prostaglandins, for digestion and rupture of the follicular wall.
C. It occurs after ferning of cervical mucus has disappeared.
D. During ovulation, the release of the ovum may take as long as 30 min.
E. On day 23 of a normal menstrual cycle the appearance of subnuclear vacuolation on endometrial biopsy strongly indicates that ovulation has occurred.

147. Testis:

A. Develops in the gonadal ridge before 7 weeks' gestation.
B. Testosterone reduces plasma luteinizing hormone (LH). Except in large doses, it has no effect on plasma follicle-stimulating hormone (FSH).
C. The first mitotic proliferation of spermatogenesis generates genetic diversity and halves the chromosome number.
D. The testes descend through the inguinal canal after birth.
E. Normal testis development requires only the presence of the *SRY* gene (sex-determining region on the Y chromosome).

148. **Testis:**
A. Testosterone synthesis in the human fetal testis begins at the eighth week of gestation, reaches a peak at 35 weeks, and then declines.
B. Most sperm are stored in the epididymis.
C. The rate of testosterone synthesis and secretion is dependent on follicle-stimulating hormone (FSH).
D. Sertoli cells lie inside the seminiferous tubules.
E. The testes are one of the sources of progesterone, oestrone and oestradiol in the male.

149. **Sperm/seminiferous tubules:**
A. The seminiferous tubules consist of Sertoli cells and primitive spermatagonia.
B. The seminiferous chords give rise to the seminiferous tubules.
C. Sperm can be found in the seminiferous tubules before puberty.
D. Spermatozoa have the power to fertilize 24 h after being implanted in the vagina.
E. Sertoli cells respond mainly to follicle-stimulating hormone (FSH).

150. **General endocrine:**
A. Oestrogens have a 21-carbon-based nucleus.
B. Tanycytes are specialized ependymal cells with ciliated borders which line the third ventricle over the site of the median eminence.
C. Steroid receptors are made up of two steroid binding units and one non-binding subunit.
D. Prolactin is encoded by a single gene on the long arm of chromosome 6.
E. Follicle-stimulating hormone (FSH) is a polypeptide hormone.

151. **General endocrine:**
A. Adrenocorticotrophic hormone (ACTH) is a polypeptide with a molecular weight of 45 000 daltons.
B. Protein hormones are stored by the Golgi apparatus.
C. Sex hormone-binding globulin (SHBG) binds testosterone with an affinity 50 000 times greater than that of albumin.
D. Androgens have a 19-carbon-based nucleus.
E. Human chorionic gonadotrophin (hCG) acts through a different receptor than luteinizing hormone (LH).

152. **Steroid hormones:**
A. Steroid hormones are based on a nucleus of three, six-carbon rings.
B. Sex hormones are secreted by the adrenal medulla.
C. Serum levels of sex hormone-binding globulin (SHBG) are increased by oestradiol and testosterone.
D. All steroid hormones are synthesized from acetate or acetyl co-enzyme A.
E. There is a delay of up to 2 days between the peak level of a steroid in blood and the peak of the conjugate in urine.

153. Oestrogen:
A. Stimulates the growth and activity of the mammary gland and the endometrium.
B. Is derived from cholesterol.
C. Some 80 percent of oestrogen is bound to albumin.
D. In pregnancy, oestriol is the predominant oestrogen.
E. Increases the clotting factors VII, VIII, IX and X.

154. Oestrogen:
A. Is responsible for the growth of pubic hair in the female at puberty.
B. Causes an increase in blood and urine levels of calcium.
C. Is active during pregnancy.
D. Causes deposition of glycogen in vaginal epithelium.
E. Reduces the number of progesterone receptors in the endometrium.

155. Androgen:
A. The secretion rate of dehydroepiandrosterone sulphate ($DHEA.SO_4$) is greater than that of testosterone.
B. Dihydrotestosterone is less potent than testosterone.
C. Excess androgen in prepubertal boys can lead to precocious pseudopuberty.
D. Secretion of adrenal androgen is controlled by adrenocorticotrophic hormone (ACTH).
E. Dihydrotestosterone induces and maintains differentiation of male somatic tissues.

156. Testosterone:
A. Is responsible for the development of the Wolffian duct in the male.
B. In the female, testosterone is largely derived from conversion of androstenedione.
C. Causes sodium and water retention.
D. Depresses pituitary secretion of luteinizing hormone (LH).
E. Administration increases sex hormone-binding globulin (SHBG) levels.

157. Gonadotrophin releasing hormone (GnRH):
A. Oestrogen exerts inhibitory effects at the level of the hypothalamus by increasing GnRH pulsatile secretion.
B. Has both autocrine and paracrine functions throughout the body.
C. Has been found in the ovary.
D. The cells that produce GnRH originate from the olfactory area of the brain.
E. GnRH agonists cannot be administered intramuscularly.

158. Testosterone:
A. Is a polypeptide.
B. When it is administered systemically, it stimulates spermatogenesis.
C. It is responsible for the involution of the Müllerian system in the female.
D. Induces secondary sexual characteristics in the male.
E. Is secreted by the adrenal medulla.

159. Thyroid gland:
A. The amount of free (non-protein-bound) thyroxine (T_4) in the plasma is four times greater than the amount of free tri-iodothyronine (T_3).
B. Thyroid hormone decreases the dissociation of oxygen from haemoglobin by increasing red cell 2,3-diphosphoglycerate (DPG).
C. Over-treatment of the pregnant mother with antithyroid drugs may result in cretinism.
D. Reverse T_3 is increased in severe illness.
E. Thyroid-stimulating hormone (TSH) levels are increased during normal pregnancy.

160. Gonadotrophin-releasing hormone (GnRH):
A. GnRH is derived by cleavage from a larger precursor called prepro-GnRH.
B. It is a small peptide comprising 10 amino acids.
C. It has a long half-life of 12–18 h.
D. Prolactin diminishes the secretion of GnRH.
E. The pulses of GnRH are directly under the influence of a dual catecholaminergic system.

161. Thyroid gland:
A. It develops as a thickening of the roof of the pharynx.
B. Deficiency of the thyroid hormones leads to anovulation associated with increased luteinizing hormone (LH) levels.
C. In the fetus, thyroxine (T_4) can be detected in the serum from 32 weeks onwards.
D. During pregnancy, there is a marked increase in secreted levels of thyroxine-binding globulin (TBG).
E. Thyroglobulin is a glycoprotein of molecular weight 660 000 daltons.

162. Progesterone:
A. Pregnanediol glucuronide is the major metabolite of secreted progesterone.
B. Some 80 per cent of circulating progesterone binds to the corticosteroid-binding globulin.
C. The maximum secretion of progesterone from the corpus luteum occurs 8 days after the luteinizing hormone (LH) surge.
D. The two forms of progesterone receptor are expressed by two different genes.
E. Large doses of progesterone produce natriuresis.

163. Progesterone:
A. Is a thermogenic hormone.
B. During the luteal phase, progesterone blocks the positive feedback effect of oestradiol.
C. The progesterone receptor is increased by progestins.
D. During pregnancy, progesterone inhibits the stimulatory effect of oestrogen until term.
E. Is rapidly metabolized by the liver, and approximately 20 per cent is excreted in the urine as sodium pregnanediol glucuronide.

164. Ovarian follicle:
A. At the beginning of a normal menstrual cycle, five to ten follicles become gonadotrophin-dependent and commence rapid growth.
B. The primordial follicles and their oocytes may stay in the first meiotic prophase for up to 50 years.
C. Peripheral cells of the ovarian follicle have more luteinizing hormone (LH) receptors.
D. The cells of the theca externa of the follicle are the primary source of oestrogen.
E. Ovarian cysts can occasionally be detected in fetuses by ultrasonography.

165. The corpus luteum:
A. Due to the effect of follicle-stimulating hormone (FSH) shortly after ovulation, the ruptured follicle will change to become the corpus luteum.
B. If pregnancy does not occur, the corpus luteum degenerates approximately 4 days before the next menses.
C. Luteinization is a process in which fluid rich in carotene is deposited within the cytoplasm of granulosa and theca interna cells, giving the characteristic yellow colour.
D. Mainly produces oestrogen.
E. May secrete oxytocin and inhibin.

166. General endocrine:
A. Steroid hormone receptors are located on the cell wall.
B. Human placental lactogen (hPL), both chemically and biologically, is 90 per cent similar to growth hormone (GH).
C. Progesterone has a 21-carbon-based nucleus.
D. Paracrine communication describes the way hormones and growth factors reach cells via the circulating blood.
E. Oestrogen receptors have a long half-life.

167. Antibiotics during pregnancy:
A. Aminoglycosides may cause auditory or vestibular damage, especially in the first trimester.
B. Chloramphenicol may cause 'grey baby syndrome'.
C. Tetracycline may cause dental discoloration if taken in the first trimester.
D. Metronidazole in therapeutic doses is relatively safe during pregnancy.
E. Erythromycin is safe during pregnancy.

168. Antibiotics:
A. Metronidazole given by the rectal route is as effective as when given by the intravenous route.
B. Streptomycin is nephrotoxic.
C. Aminoglycosides are effective against anaerobes.
D. Ampicillin may potentiate the anticoagulant effect of warfarin.
E. Erythromycin has an antibacterial spectrum identical to that of penicillin. Therefore, it may be used as an alternative for the penicillin-allergic patient.

169. Antibiotics:
A. Rifampicin increases the risk of neonatal bleeding in the third trimester.
B. Prolonged use of erythromycin may cause cholestatic jaundice.
C. Chloramphenicol has a wide range of activity.
D. Coxacillin is effective only against Gram-positive micro-organisms.
E. Tetracycline is the treatment of choice for *Chlamydia*.

170. Antiviral drugs:
A. Zidovudine eliminates the HIV virus.
B. Inosine pranobex enhances the B-cell response to many viruses, including herpes and HIV.
C. High levels of beta-interferon are found in the amniotic fluid and in the placenta.
D. Acyclovir prevents DNA synthesis.
E. Amantadine has a deleterious effect on breast-feeding.

171. Antiviral drugs:
A. Amantadine is effective against the HIV virus.
B. Acyclovir is a teratogenic drug.
C. Alpha-interferon is produced by the leukocytes.
D. Anaemia is a common side effect of zidovudine.
E. Idoxuridine is effective only if taken orally.

172. Local anaesthesia:
A. Local anaesthesia combined with adrenaline should be avoided in patients taking tricyclic antidepressants.
B. The total dose of adrenaline combined with local anaesthesia should not exceed 50 mg in a single operation.
C. Bupivacaine is highly protein-bound.
D. Convulsions which are a side effect of systemic absorption of lignocaine can be controlled with thiopentone and adequate oxygenation.
E. Mepivacaine, like other anaesthetics, causes vasodilatation.

173. General anaesthesia:
A. Repeated use of halothane can lead to liver damage.
B. Bone marrow depression is common after extended use of nitrous oxide.
C. Thiopental sodium is a safe anaesthetic agent for porphyria.
D. Suxamethonium has a nicotine-like action at the receptor on the endplate.
E. Thiopental sodium has no analgesic properties.

174. Regional anaesthesia:
A. Bupivacaine is the drug most widely used in epidural anaesthesia.
B. Epidural block is very useful in the management of patients with antepartum haemorrhage.
C. Spinal anaesthesia may be complicated by maternal respiratory difficulties.
D. Epidural anaesthesia may lead to a higher rate of forceps delivery.
E. Headache is more common in epidural than spinal anaesthesia.

175. Antidepressant drugs:
A. Tricyclic antidepressants may greatly potentiate the pressor effect of tyramine.
B. Serotonin uptake inhibitors such as fluoxetine (Prozac) have fewer side effects than the tricyclics.
C. Tricyclic antidepressants may cause tachycardia and irritability in the neonate.
D. Antidepressant drugs are effective in the treatment of mild depression.
E. Tricyclic antidepressants can cause convulsions.

176. Antidepressant drugs:
A. Amitriptyline can cause sudden death.
B. Fluoxetine (Prozac) is the only antidepressant that is safe to be used in children.
C. Imipramine can lead to urine retention and constipation.
D. Anaesthetics given during imipramine therapy may increase the risk of arrhythmias and hypotension.
E. Amitriptyline can cause galactorrhoea.

177. Drugs affecting glucose metabolism:
A. Biguanides should not be used in patients with even mild renal impairment.
B. Biguanides such as metformin reduce elevated blood glucose levels in diabetics and do not cause hypoglycaemia.
C. Insulin is a steroid hormone.
D. Sulphonylureas do not cross the placenta.
E. Insulin circulates in its free state in the blood.

178. Drugs affecting glucose metabolism:
A. Insulin stimulates RNA synthesis in the nucleus.
B. Glucagon increases the synthesis of glycogen.
C. Adrenaline inhibits the breakdown of hepatic glycogen.
D. Insulin is inactivated by the gastro-intestinal enzymes.
E. Glucagon can not be used in the treatment of hypoglycaemic coma.

179. Drugs acting on the thyroid gland:
A. Propylthiouracil (PTU) blocks the incorporation of iodine into tyrosine.
B. Perchlorate prevents the uptake of iodide by the follicular cells in the thyroid gland.
C. Bone marrow depression is a recognized side effect of carbimazole.
D. PTU appears in breast milk in an insignificant amount.
E. Intravenous L-thyroxine is the treatment of choice in hypothyroid coma.

180. Drugs acting on the thyroid gland:
A. Thyroid-stimulating hormone (TSH) is synthetized and released from the thyroid gland.
B. Propylthiouracil (PTU) crosses the placenta in high doses and may cause fetal goitre.
C. Anginal pain is a recognized side effect of liothyronine (Tertroxin).
D. Carbimazole is contra-indicated in breastfeeding.
E. Propranolol does cross the placenta.

181. The following treatment/drugs are correctly coupled with their teratogenic effects:
A. Irradiation – Leukaemia.
B. Warfarin – Gastroschisis.
C. Phenytoin – Cleft palate.
D. Quinine – Hypoplasia of optic nerves.
E. Aminoglycosides – Deafness.

182. Regarding the femoral vessels and nerve:
A. The origin of the femoral nerve is L2–L4.
B. The femoral nerve enters the femoral sheath and lies lateral to the femoral vessels.
C. Branches of femoral artery include the inferior epigastric artery.
D. The femoral artery lies medial to the femoral nerve.
E. The femoral artery is a continuation of the external iliac artery after passing over the inguinal ligament.

183. The femoral canal:
A. Is about 1.3 cm (1/2 inch) long.
B. Its lower opening is referred to as the femoral ring.
C. The femoral canal is the term used to name the small medial compartment for the lymphatics.
D. It contains fatty connective tissue, all the efferent lymph vessels from the deep inguinal lymph nodes, and one of the superficial inguinal lymph nodes.
E. The lower end of the canal is normally closed.

184. Teratogenic agents include:
A. Methyldopa.
B. Diethylstilboestrol.
C. Quinine.
D. Phenytoin.
E. Thalidomide.

185. The following drugs should be avoided during lactation:
A. Amantadine.
B. Androgen.
C. Co-amoxiclav.
D. Captopril.
E. Frusemide.

186. Teratogenic agents:
A. Warfarin cannot cross the placenta.
B. Lithium may cause cardiac abnormalities.
C. Chlorpheniramine may cause neonatal hypoglycaemia.
D. Aminoglycosides may cause cardiac abnormalities.
E. Ranitidine should be avoided during pregnancy.

187. Anticancer agents:
A. Vinblastine is an antimetabolite.
B. Alkylating agents cause structural damage to chromosomes at the time of replication during interphase.
C. Methotrexate therapy might lead to a peripheral neuritis.
D. Vincristine binds to tubulin and causes metaphase arrest.
E. Androgens have a beneficial effect in certain mammary gland cancers.

188. Anticancer agents:
A. Cyclophosphamide is used in the treatment of rheumatoid arthritis.
B. Busulfan is an alkylating agent.
C. Platinum derivatives cause cross-linkage of complementary DNA strands, thus preventing replication.
D. Fluorouracil (5-FU) inhibits folic reductase.
E. Methotrexate can lead to ovarian failure.

189. Drugs acting on the uterus:
A. Myometrial hypertrophy is encouraged by oestrogen.
B. Ergometrine, if given intramuscularly, acts within 3 min.
C. Oxytocin in high doses may lead to hypernatraemia.
D. Ritodrine is a beta-2-adrenoreceptor antagonist.
E. Ergometrine has anti-emetic properties.

190. Drugs acting on the uterus:
A. Ergometrine is an oxytocic.
B. Prostaglandin $F_{2\alpha}$ may lead to elevation of blood pressure.
C. Oxytocin is a nonapeptide hormone.
D. Mifepristone is an antiprogestogenic steroid.
E. Ergometrine has a greater effect on the uterus at term than in early pregnancy.

191. Drugs acting on the uterus:
A. Dinoprostone is preferable to oxytocin for induction of labour in women with intact membranes.
B. Prostaglandin inhibitors (e.g. indomethacin) are used to suppress premature labour.
C. Atropine has no direct effect on the uterus.
D. At term, the dose of syntocinon required to induce labour is 0.5–15 mU/min.
E. Oxytocin is produced by the anterior pituitary gland.

192. Contraception and sex hormones:
A. Oral testosterone is effective in the treatment of male hypogonadism.
B. Ovulation is inhibited by medroxyprogesterone acetate.
C. Intra-uterine device insertion is less effective than the hormonal methods of emergency contraception.
D. The oral contraceptive pill is free from central nervous system side effects.
E. Combined oral contraceptives reduce the risk of ovarian and endometrial cancers.

193. Contraception and sex hormones:
A. The effectiveness of the combined oral contraceptive pill is increased by rifampicin.
B. Combined oral contraceptives increase the incidence of premenstrual tension.
C. Spironolactone, an aldosterone antagonist which is used as a diuretic, is also an anti-androgen.
D. Previous venous thrombosis is an absolute contra-indication to the use of combined oral contraceptives.
E. Cyproterone acetate can cause hirsutism.

194. Contraception and sex hormones:
A. Mifepristone is antiprogestogenic.
B. Cyproterone acetate leads to increased levels of cortisol in the blood.
C. Thyroid-binding globulin plasma concentration is reduced in women using the combined oral contraceptive pill.
D. Regular menstrual cycles and fertility return to normal within 6 months of the last progestogen injection (Depo-Provera®).
E. Progestogens are contra-indicated in patients with porphyria.

195. Contraception and sex hormones:
A. There is an increased incidence of ovarian cancer in the users of the combined oral contraceptive pill.
B. Conversion of cholesterol to pregnenolone is the rate-limiting step in the production of sex steroid hormones.
C. The combined oral contraceptive pill contains between 20 and 50 µg of ethinyl estradiol.
D. Progesterones have a major role in the treatment of threatened abortion.
E. Contraceptive implants (e.g. Implanon®) provide up to 5 years of continuous contraceptive efficacy.

196. Inflammation:
A. Following trauma, there may be initial vasodilatation followed by vasoconstriction.
B. A cell-free plasmatic zone adjacent to the endothelium of venules is only seen in normal cells.
C. The margination of white cells phenomenon is very characteristic of chronic inflammation.
D. One of the essential features of an abscess is a lining pyogenic membrane consisting of necrotic tissue.
E. Kinins are polypeptides.

197. Inflammation:
A. Phagocytosis is a characteristic function of plasma cells.
B. Fibrosis is a minor feature of ulcerative colitis.
C. Resolution means the complete return to normal following acute inflammation.
D. *Staphylococcus pyogenes* is the causative organism in osteomyelitis.
E. In acute inflammation, the crucial factor in formation of an inflammatory exudate is increased permeability of the vessel wall to plasma proteins.

198. Chronic inflammation:

A. Is associated with increased levels of IgG in the blood.
B. In chronic pyelonephritis there are multiple small abscesses in the renal cortex.
C. In chronic inflammation the inflammatory and healing processes proceed side by side.
D. Pyaemia is an essential feature of abscess formation.
E. Endoarteritis obliterans is the condition in which there are occlusions of medium-sized arteries by intimal proliferation.

199. Acute inflammation:

A. Fibrin forms a union between severed tissues.
B. Kinins are polypeptides which cause relaxation of smooth muscle.
C. Eosinophilia is characteristic of asthma and diphtheria.
D. Prostacyclin is responsible for increased capillary permeability.
E. The monocyte cells are the first cells to emigrate through the endothelial gaps.

200. Syphilis:

A. Syphilitic chancre is painful.
B. Chancre usually appears on the genital region 2–4 weeks after infection.
C. The Wasserman reaction (WR) is a specific test.
D. Aortitis is a feature of secondary syphilis.
E. Is caused by a spirochaete.

201. Chemical mediators concerned in production of an inflammatory response include:

A. Globulin permeability factor.
B. Bradykinin.
C. 5-Hydroxytryptamine.
D. Plasma kinins.
E. Histamine.

202. Amyloidosis:

A. Is a type of coagulative necrosis.
B. Granulation tissue is a feature of amyloidosis.
C. The amyloid deposits lie around blood vessels.
D. Renal failure is the terminal manifestation.
E. Rarely affects the liver.

203. Tuberculosis:

A. Is characterized by a cellular reaction which includes siderocytes.
B. *Mycobacterium tuberculosis* is destroyed by drying.
C. *Mycobacterium tuberculosis* is a Gram-positive bacterium.
D. The bacterium *Mycobacterium tuberculosis* is always penicillin-sensitive.
E. Tuberculosis of the genital tract is usually a blood-borne infection.

204. Inflammation:
A. The exudate of acute inflammation contains more than 3 per cent protein.
B. C-reactive protein (CRP) is produced in the liver in response to inflammation elsewhere in the body.
C. Histamine stimulates gastric secretion.
D. An acute inflammatory exudate does not clot.
E. Serotonin is released from the red blood cells.

205. Wound healing:
A. Is delayed by the presence of dead tissue.
B. Collagen is a polysaccharide.
C. Nerve cells can regenerate.
D. Healing by primary intention is fast and leaves a small, neat scar.
E. Collagen has a high content of hydroxyproline and proline.

206. Wound healing:
A. Zinc is an essential factor in wound healing.
B. The acute inflammation phase is followed by a demolition phase.
C. The healing process is fastest in the trunk and limbs.
D. The limit of epithelial in-growth from the margins of a wound is 5 mm.
E. Is delayed by the presence of infection.

207. The metabolic response to injury:
A. The main source of energy is liver glycogen.
B. Potassium excretion in urine is increased.
C. There is an increase in insulin secretion.
D. The specific gravity of the urine is increased.
E. Liver glycogen is mobilized.

208. The metabolic response to injury:
A. There is an increased release of vasopressin.
B. Replacement of plasma proteins takes 2–3 weeks.
C. Nitrogen excretion is increased.
D. Fatty acid levels in blood are increased.
E. There is an increased output of adrenaline and noradrenaline in the urine.

209. Shock:
A. Is associated with bradycardia.
B. Endotoxic shock can cause kidney damage only by direct damage to renal epithelium.
C. Tissue hypoxia leads to metabolic acidosis.
D. Hypovolaemic shock follows haemorrhage of 5 per cent or more of blood volume.
E. The metabolic rate is reduced.

210. Shock:
A.   Bacteraemic shock is improved by massive doses of steroids.
B.   In anaphylactic shock, histamine is released from the mast cells.
C.   Cholera infection can cause hypovolaemic shock.
D.   There is a reduction in body temperature.
E.   Endotoxic shock is caused by polypeptide toxins.

211. The following viruses are correctly coupled with their associated tumour:
A.   Epstein–Barr virus: Burkitt's lymphoma.
B.   Epstein–Barr virus: nasopharyngeal tumours.
C.   Herpes type I: carcinoma of the cervix.
D.   Human papillomavirus: uterine fibroid.
E.   Hepatitis B: ovarian carcinoma.

212. The following are pre-cancerous lesions:
A.   Ectopic testis.
B.   Ulcerative colitis.
C.   Polyposis coli.
D.   Paget's disease of the breast.
E.   Neurofibromatosis.

213. Abnormal tissue growth and pre-invasive lesions:
A.   Vulval intra-epithelial neoplasia (VIN) is associated with human papillomavirus (HPV), especially in younger women.
B.   Vaginal intra-epithelial neoplasia (VAIN) usually presents with vaginal pain.
C.   Dyskaryosis is a histological term which refers to an abnormality of an individual cell.
D.   Dysplasia is a histological diagnosis which describes abnormalities of epithelium.
E.   HPV type 16, 18, 31, 36 are found in 30 per cent of invasive cervical cancers.

214. The following are examples of cancers related to environmental or occupation influences:
A.   Bone: wood workers.
B.   Gut: nitrosamines.
C.   Scrotum: mineral oil.
D.   Nasal sinus: aflatoxin.
E.   Lung: smoking.

215. Tumour:
A.   Rhabdomyoma is a benign tumour.
B.   Breast cancer has a high incidence in Japan.
C.   Teratoma of the testis is commonest between the ages of 50 and 60 years.
D.   Uterine fibroids are present in at least 20 per cent of women over the age of 35 years.
E.   Seminoma is a benign neoplasm.

216. Tumour:
A. Breast cancer occurs in about 10 per cent of men.
B. Carcinoma of the prostate usually occurs before the age of 40 years.
C. Adrenocorticotrophic hormone (ACTH) is produced by the Oat cell carcinoma of the lung.
D. Nasopharyngeal carcinoma is more common among woodworkers.
E. Bladder cancer is related to *Schistosoma mansonii* infection.

217. Tumour:
A. Conn's tumour produces angiotensin.
B. Carcinoid tumour is associated with pulmonary hypertension.
C. Cushing's disease is associated with increased secretion of adrenocorticotrophic hormone (ACTH).
D. Dysgerminoma is radiosensitive.
E. Carcinoma of the prostate leads to osteolytic bone metastases.

218. The following tumours are malignant:
A. Phaeochromocytoma.
B. Osteosarcoma.
C. Seminoma.
D. Lipoma.
E. Fibroma.

219. The following tumours and products are commonly associated:
A. Basophil adenoma: corticotrophin (ACTH).
B. Endodermal sinus tumours: human chorionic gonadotrophin (hCG).
C. Phaeochromocytoma: gastrin.
D. Carcinoid tumour: heparin.
E. Granulosa cell tumour: oestrogen.

220. Tumour:
A. There are both cytotrophoblastic and syncytial elements in complete hydatidiform mole.
B. The bladder base is the commonest site of bladder carcinoma.
C. Melanomas contain melanin derived from glycine.
D. Seminoma is a benign neoplasm.
E. Acanthoma arises from fibroblasts.

221. Tumour:
A. Fast-growing tumours have a doubling time of 20–24 h.
B. Translocation of oncogenes has been shown in carcinoma of the ovary.
C. Malignant tumours rarely invade the surrounding tissues.
D. Slow-growing tumours have a doubling time of 100 days.
E. In malignant tumours the number of chromosomes may be decreased.

222. Immunoglobulin:
A. Antiviral activity is provided mainly by IgA antibody.
B. Immunoglobulins G are produced by T helper cells.
C. All immunoglobulins are gamma-globulins.
D. Immunoglobulin G (IgG) chains are coded for by adjacent genes on the same chromosome.
E. Immunoglobulin M (IgM) is a cryoglobulin.

223. Immunology:
A. Immunoglobulin G of fetal origin is secreted after birth.
B. Immunoglobulin G is produced in similar amounts in all individuals exposed to the same stimulus.
C. Immunoglobulin M does not cross the placenta.
D. Immunoglobulin M is produced in the primary immune response.
E. Immunoglobulin formation requires complement.

224. Immunology:
A. The basic immunoglobulin molecule consists of three peptide chains.
B. The plasma concentration of IgA is 1000 mg/dL.
C. The main function of IgM is complement fixation.
D. The memory B cells secrete large quantities of antibodies into the general circulation.
E. IgG freely crosses the placental barrier.

225. Immunoglobulin:
A. The basic component of each immunoglobulin contains four polypeptides chains.
B. The constant region of heavy chain forms an antigen-binding site.
C. Immunoglobulins are produced by T cells.
D. The main function of immunoglobulin E is release of histamine from basophils and mast cells.
E. Immunoglobulin A is the major immunoglobulin of the external secretions.

226. Haemolytic disease of newborn:
A. About 50 per cent of Rh-negative individuals are sensitized (develop an anti-Rh titre) by transfusion of Rh-positive blood.
B. Could be caused by anti-Kell antibodies.
C. Fetal haemoglobin and Coomb's test should be checked on cord blood if the mother is rhesus positive with anti-Kell antibodies.
D. In rhesus isoimmunization the level of maternal IgM is high in the cord blood.
E. Without prophylaxis, haemolytic disease occurs in about 17 per cent of Rh-positive fetuses born to Rh-negative mothers who have previously been pregnant with Rh-positive fetuses.

227. Haemolytic disease of the newborn:
A. It is reduced if there is parental ABO incompatibility.
B. Factor II, VII, IX and X are vitamin K-dependent.
C. Platelet counts are reduced.
D. Could be due to anti-Lewis antibodies.
E. The direct Coombs' test detects the presence of free immunoglobulin in serum.

228. Immunology and pregnancy:
A. IgG decreases in pregnancy.
B. Helper T lymphocytes are increased in number in normal pregnancy.
C. Maternal IgG has no harmful effect on the fetus.
D. Fetal IgM is derived from maternal blood.
E. IgD is increased in pregnancy.

229. Immunology:
A. Macrophage activated factor is released by activated helper T cells.
B. Gamma interferon increases the cytotoxicity of natural killer (NK) cells.
C. Interleukin-1 is derived exclusively from monocytes.
D. Immunoglobulin D is increased in normal pregnancy.
E. T lymphocytes (T cells) play a major role as antigen-reactive cells and effect cell-mediated immunity.

230. Immunology:
A. Immunoglobulin A is present in colostrum.
B. Helper T cells are essential in order for B cells to produce full activation and antibody formation.
C. The genes of the major histocompatibility complex (MHC) are located on the short arm of human chromosome 6.
D. Lymphokines are produced by lymphocytes.
E. Most of the receptors on T cells are made up of alpha and beta polypeptides units.

231. The complement system:
A. The central component between the two pathways is C5.
B. The complement system consists of a set of insoluble serum proteins.
C. It mediates the cell killing effects of innate immunity as well as acquired immunity.
D. The alternative pathway is activated by an antigen–antibody interaction.
E. C3b can become a C3 convertase which amplifies the system.

232. Adrenal cortex:
A. Comprises two morphologically distinct regions.
B. During fetal life, the fetal adrenal cortex represents 20 per cent of the gland.
C. The ratio of secreted cortisol to corticosterone is approximately 1:17.
D. The zona fasciculata produces aldosterone.
E. After hypophysectomy, the three zones begin to atrophy.

233. The human rectum:
A. Is about 12 cm (5 inches) long.
B. Has no mesentery.
C. Is covered anteriorly by peritoneum along its whole length.
D. Has a blood supply from the terminal branches of the superior mesenteric artery.
E. Has appendices epiplicae.

234. Regarding the anterior abdominal wall:
A. All lymphatic drainage occurs into the inguinal nodes.
B. Cutaneous branches from the superior and inferior epigastric arteries supply the area near the midline.
C. Branches from the intercostal and lumbar arteries supply the flanks.
D. Incisions across the natural lines of cleavage heal as a narrow scar.
E. The external oblique, the internal oblique and the rectus abdominis are the muscles of the anterior and lateral abdominal wall.

235. The perineal body:
A. Is called the central perineal tendon.
B. Lies in front of the vagina.
C. The external anal sphincter inserts into it.
D. Is mainly formed of fibrous tissue.
E. Puborectalis muscle contributes to it.

236. The female breast:
A. Is ectodermal in origin.
B. Has a lymphatic connection between both sides.
C. Is made up of 30–40 units of glandular tissue.
D. Receives sympathetic innervation.
E. Malignancy spreads to the vertebrae through lymphatic channels.

237. The following are true about the vulva:
A. The Bartholin's glands are the homologues of Cowper's gland in the male.
B. The vestibule lies between the hymen and the labia majora.
C. The skin of the vulva is drained into the medial group of superficial inguinal lymph nodes.
D. The Bartholin's gland lies deep to the bulbo-spongiosus muscle.
E. The skin of the vestibule is stratified squamous epithelium without hair follicles.

238. The adult female breast:
A. Is an example of an exocrine gland.
B. Starts to develop before the menarche.
C. Has abundant fatty tissue beneath the areola.
D. Shows alveolar proliferation in man due to progesterone.
E. Requires thyroxine for full development.

239. The labia minora:

A. Are derived from the same embryological structure as the labia majora.
B. Contain sebaceous glands.
C. The epithelium is keratinized on both sides.
D. Are more sensitive, having more nerve endings than the labia majora.
E. Have lymphatic drainage to the superficial and deep subinguinal nodes.

240. Regarding the pituitary gland:

A. The anterior pituitary is of ectodermal origin.
B. It increases in weight during pregnancy.
C. It secretes releasing factors.
D. It has acidophil cells which secrete adrenocorticotrophic hormone (ACTH).
E. It has a rich blood supply.

Answers

1.
A. **False.** It is fat-soluble.
B. **True.** Also in cases of pancreatic disease where there is pancreatic lipase deficiency.
C. **True.**
D. **False.** Vitamins are organic dietary constituents necessary for life, health and growth that do not function by supplying the body with energy.
E. **True.**

2.
A. **False.** It is water-soluble.
B. **False.** It is absorbed mainly in the lower ileum, aided by gastric intrinsic factor.
C. **True.**
D. **True.**
E. **True.** The source is mainly from animal foodstuffs; vegetables alone are an inadequate source.

3.
A. **True.**
B. **False.**
C. **True.** Tetrahydrofolate is essential for both purine and pyrimidine biosynthesis.
D. **False.** The normal Western diet contains 500–700 μg per day, of which 10–100 per cent may be lost in cooking.
E. **False.**

4.
A. **False.** Citrus food and leafy green vegetables are rich in vitamin C, while animal sources contain only traces.
B. **True.**
C. **False.** The eye and the adrenal glands contain large quantities of vitamin C.
D. **True.**
E. **True.**

5.
A. **True.**
B. **False.** The body contains only 30 mg (the average adult requirement is 1–1.5 mg/day).
C. **True.** As with other water-soluble vitamins, vitamin B crosses the placenta by active mechanisms, which results in higher concentration in the fetus.
D. **False.** The true figure is 2.5 mg per day, and in non-pregnant adult is 2 mg per day.
E. **True.**

6.
A. False.
B. True.
C. False.   Xerophthalmia is due to vitamin A deficiency. Hypervitaminosis A is characterized by anorexia, headache, hepatosplenomegaly, patchy loss of hair and hyperostosis.
D. True.
E. False.   During pregnancy the requirement is 1000 µg per day.

7.
A. False.
B. True.
C. False.   It is absorbed from the small intestine.
D. True.
E. True.

8.
A. False.   It is present in most food.
B. False.   Proven only in animals and not in humans.
C. True.
D. False.   There is no evidence that vitamin E increases virility, or plays any role in the treatment of infertility or recurrent abortion.
E. True.

9.
A. True.
B. True.   The only exception is in pregnant patients on anti-epileptic drugs who require vitamin K in the last month of pregnancy and in newborn babies whose colons have not yet been colonized by bacteria.
C. True.
D. True.   Both are derivatives of the cyclic structure naphthoquinone.
E. False.   Although vitamin K accumulates initially in the liver, its hepatic concentration declines rapidly.

10.
A. True.
B. True.
C. True.
D. False.   It is 2000 kcal per day.
E. False.   The metabolic rate is increased after consumption of a meal that is rich in protein or fat.

11.
A. **False.** Oxidation is the combination of a substance with oxygen, or loss of hydrogen, or loss of an electron. Reduction is the reverse of this.
B. **True.**
C. **False.** It is an organic, non-protein substance.
D. **True.**
E. **True.**

12.
A. **True.**
B. **True.**
C. **False.** A change in pH has an effect on enzyme activity.
D. **True.**
E. **True.**

13.
A. **False.** Protein on average is composed of 16 per cent nitrogen and 84 per cent of carbon, hydrogen and sulphur combined.
B. **True.** Peptide chains contain 2–10 amino acid residues, while polypeptide chains contain >10 to over 100 amino acid residues.
C. **False.** The yield is 4 kcal per gram absorbed.
D. **True.**
E. **False.** In the case of pre-eclampsia, where the liver is affected, there is a further fall in albumin concentration.

14.
A. **False.** It is the end-product of purine metabolism in humans.
B. **False.** It is excreted mainly in the urine, but some is excreted in the bile.
C. **False.** It is not very soluble in body fluids.
D. **True.**
E. **True.** The clearance of uric acid is increased, but this is balanced by increased tubular reabsorption.

15.
A. **False.** The principal carbohydrate used in body metabolism is glucose.
B. **False.** Glycolysis is the process whereby glycogen is broken down to either pyruvate (aerobic metabolism) or lactate (anaerobic metabolism).
C. **False.** The pentose shunt is active in all cells of the body, including fat and RBC.
D. **True.**
E. **True.** When carbohydrate supply is limited, the body uses fats for energy. Excess acetyl CoA may be produced, which condenses to acetoacetyl-CoA, the origin of the ketone bodies.

16.
A. **True.**   Over 4000 single gene defects have been recorded. However, the disorders occur rarely due to autosomal recessive inheritance.
B. **False.**   Risks within an affected family are usually high and are calculated by knowing the mode of inheritance and details of the family pedigree.
C. **True.**
D. **True.**   For example, alpha-thalassaemia.
E. **False.**   It is more likely to arise by a new mutation than by direct inheritance.

17.
A. **True.**
B. **True.**
C. **True.** Some cases.
D. **True.**
E. **False.**

18.
A. **False.**   It is a Y-linked disorder.
B. **True.**
C. **True.**
D. **False.**   It is an autosomal dominant disorder.
E. **False.**   It is an autosomal recessive disorder.

19.
A. **True.**
B. **True.**
C. **True.**
D. **True.**
E. **True.**

20.
A. **False.**   Nuclear chromatin (Barr body) represents an inactivated X chromosome, which may be maternal or paternal in origin.
B. **False.**   It is a genetic disorder with autosomal dominant inheritance, so the karyotype is normal.
C. **True.**   The Karyotype is 47, XXY.
D. **True.**   The Karyotype is 47, trisomy 18.
E. **True.**   Other features include wide carrying angle, webbed neck, streak ovaries, primary amenorrhoea and infertility. Two-thirds of fetuses with Turner's syndrome die *in utero* and are characterized by a cystic hygroma on prenatal ultrasound. The one third that survive are usually XO mosaics.

21.

A. **True.** Banding techniques are used to distinguish chromosomes. Banding patterns show genetic polymorphism (i.e. differences between individuals), and it is sometimes possible to trace fetal autosomes to a specific parent.

B. **True.** Using quinacrine dye.

C. **True.**

D. **True.**

E. **True.**

22.

A. **True.**

B. **True.**

C. **False.** The proximal part of the mesonephric duct becomes greatly elongated and convoluted to become the epididymis.

D. **False.** During development, the mesonephros is replaced by the metanephros and disappears, except for some of its tubules which persist to form the vas deferens which drains the testis into the epididymis.

E. **True.**

23.

A. **False.** Appendix testis and utriculus masculinus are remnants of the paramesonephric duct in the male.

B. **True.**

C. **True.**

D. **True.**

E. **True.**

24.

A. **True.** In the upper strait the antero-posterior diameter is 11.5 cm and the transverse diameter is 13.6 cm.

B. **True.**

C. **True.** The antero-posterior diameter is 12.5 cm in the lower strait.

D. **True.**

E. **True.** The gynaecoid sacrum is broad, shallow and concave, as opposed to flattened, narrow and long.

25.

A. **True.**

B. **False.** The kidneys attain their adult position during the eighth week of fetal life.

C. **True.**

D. **True.**

E. **True.**

26.
A. True.
B. True.
C. False.   Increased excretion of folate.
D. True.
E. True.

27.
A. True.
B. True.
C. False.
D. True.
E. False.

28.
A. True.
B. True.
C. True.
D. True.
E. True.

29.
A. True.
B. False.
C. True.
D. False.
E. False.

30.
A. True.
B. False.
C. True.
D. False.   The tidal volume increases.
E. True.

31.
A. True.
B. True.
C. True.
D. False.   Compared with the adult, the neonate has a reduced concentration of vitamin K.
E. True.

32.
A. False.
B. False.
C. False.
D. False.
E. True.

33.
A. True.
B. True.
C. False.
D. False.
E. True.

34.
A. False.
B. True.
C. False.
D. False.
E. False.

35.
A. True.
B. True.
C. False. Fetal red blood cells are larger than maternal red blood cells.
D. True.
E. False. The concentration is 18 g/dL.

36.
A. True.
B. True.
C. False. The half-life is 6 h.
D. False. Half-life: 72 h in blood, but in the tissues it is unknown (may be 3 months).
E. False. After birth, some lymphocytes are formed in the bone marrow, but most are formed in the lymph nodes, thymus and spleen from precursor cells that originally came from the bone marrow.

37.
A. True.
B. False. Fetal haemoglobin has a low affinity for oxygen.
C. True. Surfactants are formed of a mixture of phospholipids (77%), natural lipids (13%), proteins (8%) and carbohydrates (2%).
D. True.
E. False. They decrease within 72 h prior to the spontaneous onset of labour.

38.
A. True.
B. False.   Some 68% will be within one SD, 95% will be within two SDs, and 99.73% will be within 3 SDs.
C. True.
D. False.   Non-parametric tests can be used on normal and non-normal data. Parametric tests can only be used on normal data.
E. True.   The degrees of freedom can be calculated by (number of columns minus 1)×(number of rows minus 1). Thus, for a 2×2 table, it is $(2-1)\times(2-1)=1$.

39.
A. False.   The half-life is 120 days.
B. True.
C. True.
D. False.   RBCs are non-nucleated cells as they lose their nuclei before entering the circulation.
E. False.   An adult man has 900 g of haemoglobin in the circulating blood.

40.
A. False.   So far, they are penicillin-sensitive.
B. True.
C. True.
D. False.   They produce exotoxin.
E. True.   They produce fibrinolysin, streptodornase and hyaluronidase.

41.
A. False.   Spreading infections.
B. True.
C. False.   Pharyngeal carriage rates vary with geographical location, season of the year and age group. Among school-aged children, rates of 15–20 per cent have been reported; the carriage rate among adults is considerably lower.
D. True.   They also cause acute follicular tonsillitis, quinsy, necrotizing fasciitis, infective endocarditis and puerperal sepsis.
E. True.   Group A organisms are responsible for the great majority of human streptococcal infections. Group B are the most important vaginal pathogens responsible for preterm labour, neonatal infection and puerperal sepsis.

42.
A. False.   It is arranged in clusters (punches).
B. True.
C. True.
D. False.   It is a non-spore-forming bacterium.
E. True.   Penicillinase-producing staphylococci are sensitive to: cloxacillin, cephalosporin, fucidin, clindamycin, gentamycin and flucloxacillin.

43.

A. True.

B. True.

C. True.   It also produces fibrinolysin, haemolysins, hyaluronidase and phosphatase.

D. True.

E. False. It is haemolytic on blood agar.

44.

A. False.

B. True.

C. True.   It is also found in salads and pre-cooked meat.

D. True.

E. True.   It can proliferate at low temperature (6°C or above).

45.

A. True.

B. False. It is resistant to alkaline conditions.

C. True.   In concentrations as high as 10 per cent.

D. True.

E. True.   It can cause miscarriage, stillbirth (up to 20% of cases) and neonatal death. Listeriosis occurs throughout pregnancy and should be considered when the mother has a pyrexial flu-like illness. Many cases, however, are asymptomatic.

46.

A. False. Gram-negative diplococci are seen within the cytoplasm of polymorphs.

B. True.   Treatment is with spectinomycin or cefoxitin if the gonococcus is beta-lactamase-producing, but with probencid if it is resistant to the above drugs.

C. False. It infects columnar epithelium (e.g. ectocervix) but is unable to penetrate stratified squamous epithelium (e.g. vagina); hence a cervical swab is taken to investigate suspected lower-genital tract gonorrhoea.

D. True.

E. True.   This spreads rapidly to the accessory glands (e.g. Skene's gland); in the female, it affects the urogenital tract, rectum, tonsils and pharynx.

47.

A. True.

B. False. It is acid-fast.

C. True.

D. True.

E. False. It is a Gram-negative bacillus.

48.
A. **True.**
B. **True.**
C. **False.** It is Gram-positive.
D. **False.** At birth, the vagina is sterile, but within 1–2 days the oestrogen (derived from the maternal circulation *in utero*) leads to the appearance of Döderlein's bacillus.
E. **False.** Schick's test is used to distinguish susceptible individuals from those immune to diphtheria (not diagnostic) by injecting diphtheria toxins intradermally and observing for oedema and erythema (maximal in 2–4 days) in susceptible individuals.

49.
A. **True.** The neurotoxin blocks descending inhibitory fibres in the spinal cord, which leads to the rigidity and spasm of tetanus. Tetanospasmin is a very powerful poison, while tetanolysin may cause red blood cell lysis.
B. **True.**
C. **True.** It produces a range of enzymes (including lecithinase) which cause severe tissue necrosis ('gas gangrene'), lymphocytosis and haemolysis.
D. **True.** Botulism toxin leads to a lethal form of food poisoning, 'botulinism'. It affects the cholinergic system, blocking the release of acetylcholine at the presynaptic level.
E. **True.**

50.
A. **True.**
B. **False.** Gram-negative.
C. **True.**
D. **True.**
E. **True.** Bacterial vaginosis is a non-specific infection of the vagina, characterized by a foul-smelling, fishy discharge.

51.
A. **True.** It produces an enterotoxin. Food poisoning occurs in microepidemics after ingestion of infected meat or poultry. The incubation period is 6–12 h.
B. **False.** Streptococci do not cause food poisoning. *Staphylococcus aureus* produces an enterotoxin and is the classic 'food poisoning'. It has an incubation period of 2–6 h.
C. **True.** Transmitted by infected milk. Incubation period of 3–5 days.
D. **True.** Usually associated with canned food, it produces a potent exotoxin. Incubation period of 12–36 h.
E. **True.** Usually caused by pre-cooked rice. Produces two endotoxins. The emetic type has a short incubation period of about 2 h; the diarrhoeal type has an incubation period of 6–14 h.

52.
A. **False.** It is a non-motile organism.
B. **False.** It is aerobic, and Gram-positive.
C. **False.** It is highly resistant to drying.
D. **True.** Tubercle bacillus is resistant to stains unless heated (e.g. carbol fuchsin in the Ziehl–Neelsen method); once stained, it resists decolorization by acid.
E. **False.** It grows slowly and only on complex media (Löwenstein–Jensen, containing glycerol and egg yolk) taking 6 weeks to culture.

53.
A. **True.**
B. **False.** The incubation period is 9 to 90 days.
C. **True.**
D. **True.**
E. **False.** It crosses the placenta after 16 weeks.

54.
A. **False.** Chlamydiae are non-motile and spherical.
B. **False.** It is Gram-negative (weakly).
C. **False.** Human papillomavirus (HPV) is the most common world-wide.
D. **True.** *Chlamydia* salpingitis may be associated with peritonitis and perihepatitis.
E. **True.** This condition is caused by *Chlamydia trachomatis.*

55.
A. **False.** Rubella and cytomegalovirus (CMV) (VIIIth cranial nerve).
B. **True.** Also with rubella infection.
C. **True.** Due to intracranial calcification.
D. **True.**
E. **True.** Neonatal encephalitis.

56.
A. **True.**
B. **True.**
C. **True.**
D. **True.**
E. **False.** This is an RNA-containing virus of the paramyxovirus group.

57.
A. **True.** It is a retrovirus.
B. **False.** The incubation period is 52 months (Type II > Type I, median incubation period for full clinical AIDS is 8 years).
C. **False.**
D. **True.**
E. **True.**

58.
A. True.
B. False. Non-parametric tests can be used in normally distributed data.
C. True.
D. False.
E. True.

59.
A. False. It the most frequently occurring value.
B. True.
C. True.
D. True.
E. False. Infant mortality rate is the number of infants dying during the first year per 1000 live births.

60.
A. True. This is the piezoelectric effect.
B. True. The higher the frequency, the less the depth of penetration; vaginal transducers can use higher frequencies than abdominal transducers.
C. False. Medical ultrasound uses the range of 100–500 kHz.
D. True.
E. True.

61.
A. False.
B. False.
C. False.
D. False.
E. True.

62.
A. True.
B. False. No change.
C. True.
D. True.
E. False. Will decrease.

63.
A. False. Unless there is extreme deprivation, most of the variation in fetal weight at term is accounted for by body fat.
B. True. Maternal weight gain averages 0.35 kg per week in early pregnancy, 0.45 kg per week in mid-pregnancy, and 0.35 kg per week in late pregnancy. The average total weight gain is 12.5 kg.
C. False. Meconium is present by 16 weeks and consists of desquamated intestinal cells, intestinal juices and squamous cells.
D. True.
E. False. Gallbladder motility and emptying rate are both reduced in pregnancy.

64.

A. **True.** The pH of venous blood and interstitial fluid is 7.35; intracellular pH averages 7.0.

B. **True.** The main buffer system controlling blood pH is carbonic acid/sodium bicarbonate (in cells, potassium and magnesium bicarbonate).

C. **False.** Maternal respiratory acidosis is transmitted to the fetus, as the excess carbon dioxide can cross the placenta. The placenta is not permeable to hydrogen ions; thus metabolic acidosis has less effect on the fetus.

D. **True.** As in renal failure.

E. **False.** The CO_2 level is increased.

65.

A. **False.** Units are cm H_2O.

B. **True.**

C. **True.**

D. **True.** Although some people consider 60–70cm H_2O borderline for obstruction.

E. **True.**

66.

A. **True.**

B. **True.**

C. **True.**

D. **True.**

E. **True.**

67.

A. **True.** Diagnoses based on detecting antibodies in patients' sera are retrospective. IgM antibodies may be detected earlier in the infection (7–10 days), and are usually indicative of active as opposed to past infection.

B. **False.** The sera is stored until a convalescent phase serum is available; the two sera are then tested in parallel.

C. **True.** This is an example of a precipitation reaction based on the precipitation of antigen–antibody aggregates.

D. **True.** Some viruses (e.g. influenza) have haemaglutinin molecules on their outer surface. When virus particles are mixed with red blood cells they cause haemagglutination. In the presence of a specific antibody, however, haemagglutination is inhibited.

E. **True.**

68.

A. **False.**

B. **True.** There are 32 million new cases per year world-wide.

C. **True.**

D. **True.** Commonly used specific tests are the fluorescent treponemal antibody absorption (FTA-ABS) test and the *Treponema pallidum* haemagglutination (TPHA) test.

E. **False.** It is a Gram-negative coccus: *Neisseria gonorrhoea.*

69.
A. True.
B. True.
C. True.
D. True.
E. True.

70.
A. False. This is unlikely to be of benefit.
B. False.
C. False. May be irrelevant to mucosal protection against polio.
D. False. May be harmful in hepatitis.
E. True. An IgG titre greater than 15 IU/mL is necessary.

71.
A. True.
B. False. Adaptation to low temperatures. The second method involves serial passage in cells cultured *in vitro*.
C. True.
D. False. It is the Salk vaccine.
E. False. It is, and should, only be given immediately after childbirth or when adequate contraception can be assured. However, the real risk of an infected fetus after accidental pregnancy is extremely low.

72.
A. True. However, a live attenuated vaccine is at the experimental stage.
B. True. It is inactivated by formaldehyde, like the polio 'Salk' vaccine.
C. True. This vaccine exists in two forms: the bacterium is inactivated by heat plus phenol or acetone, and is also attenuated by chemical mutagenesis.
D. False. Measles, like rubella, is a live attenuated vaccine.
E. True. Mumps virus is inactivated by passage in chick fibroblasts.

73.
A. True. Types 1–4, based on the immunological mechanism underlying the tissue-damaging reaction.
B. False. Allergic/anaphylactic, type 2 is cytotoxic.
C. True. The principal mechanism behind type 3 (immune complex-mediated) hypersensitivity involves immune complexes, complement and polymorphonuclear leukocytes (PMN). PMN are also involved in protective immunity.
D. True. T cells that have become sensitized to foreign substances.
E. True. Kidney transplantation is an example.

74.

A. **True.**

B. **True.**

C. **False.** This is a type 3 (immune complex-mediated) hypersensitivity reaction in tissues.

D. **False.** This is a type 2 (cytotoxic) hypersensitivity reaction caused by autoantibodies.

E. **False.** This is an example of autoimmunity.

75.

A. **True.** When women are in their forties, and prior to anovulation.

B. **False.** The follicular phase duration is the major determinant.

C. **False.** Inhibin levels are decreased; the decline in inhibin allows a rise in FSH. Oestradiol and LH levels are normal.

D. **True.** And a three-fold increase in LH levels.

E. **False.** The reverse is true; FSH levels are higher than LH (half-lives are about 30 min for LH and 4 h for FSH).

76.

A. **True.** With the disappearance of follicles and oestrogen, the elevated gonadotrophins drive the remaining stromal tissue in the ovary to a level of increased testosterone production.

B. **True.** Most of which is derived from peripheral conversion of oestrone.

C. **False.** At night, when a woman is often awakened from sleep.

D. **True.**

E. **False.** The flush coincides with a surge of LH (not FSH) and is preceded by a subjective prodromal awareness that a flush is beginning.

77.

A. **True.** Oestrogen therapy improves the quality of sleep, decreasing the time to onset of sleep.

B. **True.** The bone of the spinal column constitutes a honeycomb structure providing greater surface area per unit volume.

C. **True.**

D. **False.** Up to 5 per cent of trabecular bone and 1–1.5 per cent of total bone mass loss will occur per year after the menopause. This accelerated loss will continue for 10–15 years.

E. **True.**

78.

A. **False.** The long half-life of hCG is 24 h as compared to 2 h for LH – a 10-fold difference that is due mainly to the greater sialic acid content of hCG.

B. **False.** The bonds are non-covalent.

C. **True.** The a-subunits in these glycoprotein hormones are identical, encoded for by a single gene on chromosome 6.

D. **True.**

E. **True.** Virtually all normal human tissues produce the intact hCG molecule. hCG is secreted in a pulsatile fashion from the pituitary. However, hCG produced at sites other than the placenta has little or no carbohydrate, and therefore it has a very short half-life and is rapidly cleared from the circulation. The level rarely reaches the sensitivity of the usual modern assay.

79.

A. **True.**   .

B. **False.** This maximal level is reached at 8–10 weeks' gestation. hCG levels decrease to about 10 000–20 000 IU/L by 18–20 weeks.

C. **False.** hCG remains at 10 000–20 000 IU/L until term.

D. **True.**

E. **True.**

80.

A. **True.** It is secreted by the syncytiotrophoblast cells of the placenta.

B. **False.** The half-life is very short (15 min), hence it is used as an index of placental function.

C. **False.** Although very similar in structure, it has only 3 per cent of hGH somatotrophin activity.

D. **True.** Two genes encode for hGH and three for hPL; however, only two of the hPL genes are active in the placenta, each producing the same hPL hormone.

E. **False.** Blood levels of hPL are increased with hypoglycaemia and decreased with hyperglycaemia.

81.

A. **True.** In the second half of pregnancy hPL is a major force in the diabetogenic effects of pregnancy characterized by peripheral insulin resistance and hyperinsulinaemia.

B. **True.**

C. **True.** It also stimulates insulin-like growth factor-1 (IGF-1) production.

D. **False.** During fasting states, hPL stimulates lipolysis, leading to an increase in circulating free fatty acids for utilization by the mother. Glucose and amino acids are conserved for the fetus. With sustained fasting, maternal ketone levels rise which can be utilized by the fetus – unlike free fatty acids, which do not cross the placenta.

E. **True.** The Barker hypothesis is based on a series of reports from the Medical Research Council unit in Southampton. It has shown that there is a strong link between fetal problems (such as low birthweight) and problems in adult life (such as cardiovascular disease and diabetes).

82.

A. **True.**

B. **False.** They are associated with oligohydramnios.

C. **True.** There is good evidence that they can cause intra-uterine growth retardation (IUGR), oligohydramnios and neonatal anuria. Renal failure and death may occur when given in later pregnancy.

D. **True.** If possible, and certainly by the twelfth week of gestation.

E. **True.**

83.

A. **True.** Long-term follow-up of children exposed *in utero* has demonstrated normal development up to the age of 8 years.

B. **False.** The dose is 1–3 g per day, given in two to four divided doses.

C. **True.**

D. **False.** Its adverse effects on the mother are the same as those in non-pregnant individuals: for instance, somnolence or depression. These make it unsuitable for use in the puerperium.

E. **True.** It is unusual, however, to need more than one drug. An increasing need for medication to control severe hypertension must raise the suspicion not only of superimposed pre-eclampsia, but also of underlying renal problems, or the very rare occurrence of phaeochromocytoma.

84.

A. **True.**

B. **True.** Most striking when treatment is started early in the second trimester. Findings were consistent enough to conclude that beta-blockers are contra-indicated in pregnancy, except for short-term treatment in the third trimester.

C. **False.** Labetalol is a combined alpha- and beta-blocker. The alpha-blocking action causes arteriolar vasodilatation and lowers peripheral resistance, which is why labetalol is preferred in pregnancy.

D. **False.** Oxprenolol, pindolol, acebutolol and celiprolol have ISA, which reduces side effects such as cold extremities (hands and feet) and bradycardia.

E. **False.** But they can lead to a small deterioration in glucose tolerance and may interfere with metabolic and autonomic responses to hypoglycaemia.

85.
A. **False.** Significant amounts are present in breast milk but it is not known to be harmful.
B. **False.** Methyldopa is contra-indicated to avoid exacerbating post-partum depression (depression being a side effect of the drug). However, the amount secreted in breast milk is too small to affect the baby.
C. **True.** If they were used pre-conceptually or they can be used for the first time; there is also no contra-indication to beta-blockers.
D. **False.** Breast-feeding need not be restricted in patients receiving antihypertensive medication. Although excreted into breast milk, no adverse effects on breast-fed infants exposed to methyldopa, nifedipine or labetalol have been reported. Thiazide diuretics in large doses, on the other hand, may decrease or inhibit milk production.
E. **False.** Metronidazole is secreted in significant amounts in breast milk. Manufacturer advises avoiding single large doses. In practice at normal doses it appears to be safe and is widely used.

86.
A. **True.**
B. **False.** In women with SLE who conceive, 50 per cent of babies will be born alive.
C. **True.**
D. **True.** Both may cause proteinuria, oedema, thrombocytopenia and raised blood pressure, and so patients are often treated for both conditions simultaneously.
E. **True.** Or a previous pregnancy with pre-eclampsia or intra-uterine growth retardation, or both. It should be borne in mind, however, that pre-term babies whose mothers have taken aspirin are at increased risk of intracranial haemorrhage.

87.
A. **False.** This rare condition results from passively acquired maternal anti-Ro antibodies.
B. **False.** Cutaneous neonatal lupus is the most common form and appears as a self-limiting rash, usually on the face and scalp, which is exacerbated by sunlight. No treatment is required.
C. **False.** This worrying, albeit rare, condition usually develops *in utero* from about 18 weeks' gestation and causes irreversible damage.
D. **True.**
E. **False.** High-dose corticosteroids, and also plasmapheresis, have been given to the mothers once the condition is detected in the fetus, but with little success.

88.
A. **True.** This is an observation that led to the widespread use of corticosteroids in the management of this condition.
B. **True.**
C. **False.** Congenital heart block in the fetus is an exceptionally rare complication.
D. **False.** This complication is seen with penicillamine; there have been isolated case reports of cutis laxa, inguinal hernia, and joint hypermobility. Azathioprine has been associated with intra-uterine growth retardation.
E. **False.** It is contra-indicated.

89.

A. **True.**

B. **True.**   This is largely because placental thrombosis can cause placental insufficiency and first-trimester loss or intra-uterine growth retardation, and eventually intra-uterine death.

C. **True.**

D. **False.**   Such patients require 100 mg hydrocortisone intravenously at 6-hourly intervals during labour.

E. **True.**   Because of the rare occurrence of neonatal convulsions. Usual therapeutic doses of aspirin, prednisolone, hydroxychloroquine and methyldopa are all probably safe during breast-feeding. There is a theoretical risk of fetal adrenal suppression with high doses of prednisolone, but the risk is small.

90.

A. **False.**   Glandular acini and islets of Langerhans.

B. **False.**   Three types: a, b and d cells.

C. **True.**

D. **False.**   d cells produce somatostatin, b cells produce insulin.

E. **True.**

91.

A. **False.**   All diameters are absolutely greater than in the male.

B. **True.**   In the male, the sub-pubic arch is about 50–60 degrees.

C. **False.**   The sacral promontory is more prominent in the male, so that the male inlet is heart-shaped whereas the female inlet is more rounded, facilitating engagement of the fetal head.

D. **True.**

E. **False.**   The sacrum is shorter and wider in the female, and its upper part is straight.

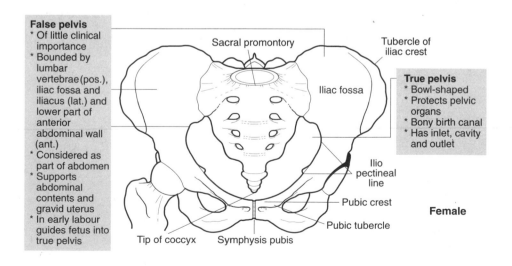

False pelvis
* Of little clinical importance
* Bounded by lumbar vertebrae (pos.), iliac fossa and iliacus (lat.) and lower part of anterior abdominal wall (ant.)
* Considered as part of abdomen
* Supports abdominal contents and gravid uterus
* In early labour guides fetus into true pelvis

Sacral promontory

Tubercle of iliac crest

Iliac fossa

True pelvis
* Bowl-shaped
* Protects pelvic organs
* Bony birth canal
* Has inlet, cavity and outlet

Ilio pectineal line

Pubic crest

Pubic tubercle

Female

Tip of coccyx   Symphysis pubis

92.

A. True.

B. True.

C. False. The two chains are joined by two disulphide bridges. Chain A comprises 21 amino acids.

D. True.

E. False. About 250 units are stored, of which about 50 units are needed per day, except in pregnancy when the insulin response to glucose is increased three-fold.

93.

A. True. It also rises to a level of 60–100 mU/mL after a standard 75-g glucose load.

B. False. The half-life is 20 min.

C. True. Which breaks the disulphide bonds between the A and B chains.

D. True. Or semisynthetically by enzymatic modification of porcine insulin.

E. False. Insulin is inactivated by gastro-intestinal enzymes and must therefore be given by injection.

94.

A. False.

B. False.

C. True.

D. True.

E. True.

95.

A. False. It consists of 29 amino acids.

B. True.

C. False. Glucagon is glycogenolytic, gluconeogenic, lipolytic and ketogenic. It is the hormone of energy release. It works in an inverse relationship with insulin: as blood levels of one fall, the other rises. When glucagon is given to treat hypoglycaemia its immediate action is rapid mobilization of glycogen (not glucose) stored in the liver. Through gluconeogenesis it creates glucose but does not mobilize it.

D. True.

E. True.

96.
A. True.
B. True.
C. True.
D. False.
E. False.

97.
A. False. Is a triangular area situated in the upper part of the medial aspect of the thigh.
B. True.
C. False. It is bounded laterally by the sartorius muscle.
D. True.
E. True.

98.
A. True.
B. True.
C. True.
D. False. The femoral triangle is bounded by the inguinal ligament superiorly.
E. True. The femoral vein is a medial relation of the femoral artery, and the artery lies on the psoas major muscle.

99.
A. True.
B. False. The sacrum consists of the five sacral vertebrae joined by bone in the adult and cartilage in the young. There are four sacral foramina communicating with the sacral canal.
C. True. The obturator foramen is bounded by the ischium and the pubis, and is occupied by a fibrous sheet, the obturator membrane. Superiorly, there is a small gap (canal) which communicates between the pelvis and the thigh and carries the obturator artery, vein and nerve.
D. False. The innominate bone consists of ilium, ischium and pubis.
E. True. It also transmits the internal pudendal vessels and nerve, the sciatic and posterior femoral cutaneous nerves, and the nerve to the quadratus femoris.

100.
A. True.
B. True. This supports the anal canal and allows it to distend during defaecation.
C. False. The internal pudendal nerves and vessels lie in the lateral walls of the fossae within the sheath.
D. False. The two fossae communicate with each other round the anal canal and are separated by the anococcygeal body, the anal canal and the perineal body.
E. True. The medial wall is formed by the sloping levator ani muscle and the anal canal.

101.
A. False. It arises from the lower eight ribs.
B. True. In addition it contains the ilioinguinal nerve and the spermatic cord (in the male).
C. True. The cutaneous nerve supply to the anterior abdominal wall is derived from the anterior rami of the lower six thoracic and the first lumbar nerves.
D. False. The pyramidalis is a triangular muscle in front of the lower part of the rectus abdominis; it is frequently absent.
E. False. The superior epigastric artery and the inferior epigastric artery with which it anastomoses both lie deep to the rectus abdominis.

102.
A. False. In the female they do not fuse.
B. True.
C. False. The blood supply is from the external and internal pudendal arteries.
D. True. As well as Meissner, Merkel and Pacini corpuscles.
E. True. The gland is palpable if infected (abscess) or obstructed (cyst).

103.
A. False. The upper four-fifths is derived from the Müllerian duct, and the lower fifth from the urogenital sinus.
B. True.
C. False. It gives rise to the distal part of the urethra and part of the vagina. These developments occur by 42 days after fertilization.
D. False. The vagina is canalized at 18 weeks' gestation.
E. False. The vaginal fluid has a higher potassium concentration than plasma, but a lower concentration of sodium.

104.

A. **False.**   If the sinovaginal bulbs fail to fuse or do not develop at all, a double vagina or atresia of the vagina, respectively results.

B. **True.**   The vaginal cells contains glycogen, which is released when the cells are exfoliated. Döderlein's bacillus, a normal inhabitant, acts upon the glycogen to produce the normal acidity of the vagina.

C. **True.**   The major nerve supply to the vagina is autonomic from the pelvic plexuses but the lower vagina has a sensory supply from the pudendal nerve.

D. **False.**   The lowest part of the vagina drains to the superficial inguinal lymph nodes, while the upper part drains to external and internal iliac and sacral nodes.

E. **False.**   The vaginal branch of the internal pudendal artery is the main blood supply to the vagina. Other sources include uterine, inferior vesical and middle rectal arteries which anastomose freely on the vaginal wall.

105.

A. **False.**   The lower portions of the Müllerian ducts fuse to form the uterus and the cervix.

B. **False.**   The uterus is also supported by the transcervical, pubocervical and uterosacral ligaments.

C. **False.**   The peritoneum covers the majority of uterus posteriorly as it covers the fundus.

D. **False.**   Secretion of angiotensin II is increased, but the vascular sensitivity to it is reduced and it is unlikely to be relevant to uterine blood flow.

E. **False.**   This occurs in up to 20 per cent of women.

106.

A. **True.**   It contains nine amino acids.

B. **True.**   Fetal oxytocin may play a role in stimulating the uterus, especially towards the end of pregnancy.

C. **True.**

D. **True.**   Oxytocin acts on the myoepithelial cells of the breast ducts, promoting milk ejection.

E. **True.**   Oxytocinase is produced by the placenta.

107.

A. **True.**   Therefore the endometrium is applied directly to the muscle.

B. **False.**   In addition there is an anastomosis with the tubal branch of the ovarian artery which contributes to the supply of the uterine fundus.

C. **True.**   At the level of the first lumbar vertebra.

D. **True.**   Same as the round ligament, which may assist in maintaining the uterus in anteversion.

E. **False.**   They are branches of the inferior epigastric plexus.

108.
A. **True.**
B. **True.** Peritoneum is reflected onto the posterior aspect of supravaginal cervix.
C. **True.** This pre-ovulatory mucus produces a ferning pattern on drying and has an alkaline pH.
D. **False.** It is lined by mucous membrane which consists of ciliated columnar epithelium in the upper two-thirds of the canal.
E. **True.** While the corpus uteri has a largely muscular structure.

109.
A. **True.** In contrast to the fallopian tubes, which are sensitive to cutting and touching.
B. **False.** The cavity of the uterus is triangular, and that of the cervix fusiform.
C. **False.** Only the lining of the endometrial cavity is shed at menstruation.
D. **True.** In addition to sacral nodes via uterosacral ligaments.
E. **True.**

110.
A. **False.** It is devoid of peritoneal cover in adults.
B. **False.** It receives its blood supply from the abdominal aorta: the ovarian artery arises at the level of the renal arteries.
C. **True.**
D. **False.** The blood drains into the inferior vena cava.
E. **False.** It drains into the para-aortic lymph nodes.

111.
A. **True.** It is an almond-shaped organ, measuring 4×2 cm (1.5×0.75 inches).
B. **True.** The scar tissue is where the old graffian follicles have ruptured.
C. **True.** The round ligament of the ovary is the remains of the upper part of the gubernaculum; that of the uterus is the remains of the lower part.
D. **True.** As well the male testes.
E. **False.** The obturator nerve, but not the artery.

Ovarian fossa

- Is bounded by:
  - Anterior: umbilical artery
  - Posterior: ureter and internal iliac artery
- Has its own mesentery, mesovarium from posterior leaf of broad ligament.
- Free surface of ovary has no peritoneal covering, only a single layered cuboidal epithelium, called the germinal epithelium.

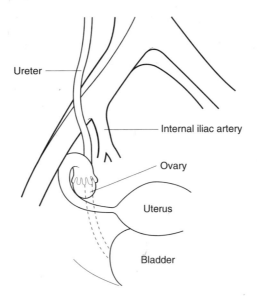

112.
A. **True.** The ovaries lie above the pelvic brim at the time of birth and do not descend until the cavity of the pelvis deepens during childhood.
B. **False.** It arises at the level of first lumbar vertebra.
C. **False.** The ureter and the internal iliac artery represent the posterior boundary of the ovarian fossa.
D. **False.** The nerve supply (the ovarian plexus) includes parasympathetic, postganglionic sympathetic and autonomic afferent fibres.
E. **False.** The enlarging uterus is more likely to pull the ovaries into the abdominal cavity.

113.
A. **True.**
B. **False.** The longitudinal fibres are only present in the part traversing the bladder wall.
C. **False.** It lies anterior to genitofemoral nerve and the external iliac vessels.
D. **False.** It has a transitional epithelium.
E. **True.** Due to pressure at the pelvic brim and high progesterone levels.

114.
A. **False.** It is 25–30 cm in length.
B. **False.** It is of mesodermal origin; it is derived by a process of budding of the caudal end of the mesonephric duct.
C. **False.** The blood supply comes from the abdominal aorta and the renal, ovarian, common and internal iliac, vesical and uterine arteries.
D. **True.** The ureter runs above the lateral fornix of the vagina, 2 cm lateral to the cervix, and then turns medially in front of the vagina.
E. **True.**

115.

A. **False.** At the upper border of the greater sciatic foramen it divides into anterior and posterior divisions.

B. **False.** The median sacral artery arises from the aorta at the point where it bifurcates into the two common iliac arteries.

C. **True.**

D. **False.** The branches of the posterior division of the internal iliac artery are iliolumbar artery, lateral sacral artery and superior gluteal artery.

E. **False.** The umbilical artery gives an artery to the vas deferens in the male and the superior vesical artery. The inferior vesicle artery originates directly from the anterior division of internal iliac artery.

116.

A. **True.** It pierces the psoas muscle to emerge from under the cover of its lateral border.

B. **False.** The lumbar plexus lies in front of the piriformis muscle and behind the ureter.

C. **False.** The femoral nerve arises from anterior divisions of L2–L4 while the obturator nerve arises from the posterior division.

D. **True.**

E. **False.** All true, except for the obturator internus muscle, which is supplied by a branch from the sacral plexus.

Origin and branches of lumbar plexus

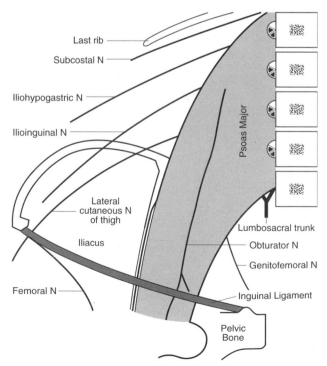

117.
A. True.
B. True.
C. False. It is a branch from lumbar plexus and it arises from L3, L4.
D. True. The sciatic nerve arises from L4 and L5; S1, S2 and S3.
E. True.

118.
A. True.
B. True. The fascia transversalis is reinforced in its medial third by the conjoint tendon.
C. False. It is a defect in the aponeurosis of the external oblique muscle.
D. True. The ilioinguinal nerve pierces the lower fibres of the internal oblique muscles to merge on the spermatic cord to pass through the superficial ring.
E. True.

119.
A. True. The aorta enters the abdomen through the aortic opening of the diaphragm in front of the twelfth thoracic vertebra.
B. True. It descends anteriorly on the bodies of the lumbar vertebrae, and in front of the fifth lumbar vertebra it divides into the two common iliac arteries.
C. True.
D. False. The external iliac artery runs along the medial border of the psoas major muscle following the pelvic brim.
E. False. The three anterior visceral branches of the aorta are the coeliac artery and the superior and inferior mesenteric arteries.

120.
A. True.
B. True. It reaches the uterus by running medially in the base of the broad ligament.
C. False. The vaginal and ovarian arteries do not enlarge during pregnancy.
D. True. Unlike the veins of the arms and legs.
E. False. The uterine vein follows the artery and drains into the internal iliac vein.

121.
A. False. The mentioned area is supplied by the superior mesenteric artery while the coeliac is the artery of the foregut.
B. True. It is 1 cm long and is surrounded by the coeliac plexus of nerves.
C. True.
D. False. The left colic artery is the larger terminal branch of the inferior mesenteric artery.
E. False. It arises from the aorta at the inferior border of the third part of the duodenum at the level of the third lumbar vertebra.

122.
A. **False.** It is about 4 cm (1.5 inches) long, and extends from the deep inguinal ring to the superficial inguinal ring.
B. **True.** The deep inguinal ring, an oval opening in the fascia transversalis, lies about 1 cm (0.5 inch) above the inguinal ligament, midway between the anterior superior iliac spine and the symphysis pubis.
C. **False.** The lacunar ligament lies at the medial end of the inguinal ligament.
D. **False.** It extends from the anterior superior iliac spine to the pubic tubercle and is the free lower border of the external oblique aponeurosis.
E. **True.** Clinically, this has value in differentiating indirect (lateral to artery) from direct (medial to artery) inguinal hernia.

123.
A. **True.** It leaves the main pelvic cavity through the greater sciatic foramen. After a brief course in the gluteal region of the lower limb it enters the perineum through the lesser sciatic foramen.
B. **False.** The inferior rectal nerve supplies the external anal sphincter, while the internal anal sphincter is supplied by the autonomic nervous system.
C. **False.** It arises from S2–S4 nerve roots.
D. **False.** They are embedded in the pudendal canal in the lateral wall of the ischiorectal fossa.
E. **False.** The pudendal nerve divides into three branches: the dorsal nerve of the clitoris, the inferior haemorrhoidal and the perineal nerves.

Pelvic fascia

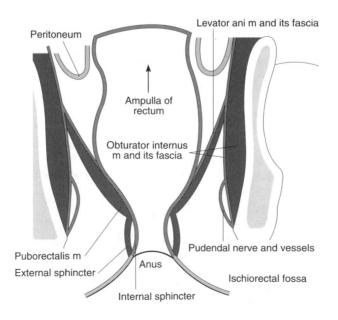

124.
A. **False.** It arises from the ventral rami of cervical nerve C3–C5.
B. **True.**
C. **True.** Branches of the phrenic nerve communicate with the coeliac plexus to supply the suprarenal, inferior vena cava and the gallbladder.
D. **True.**
E. **True.**

125.
A. **False.** The two fossae communicate with each other around the anal canal, and are separated by the anococcygeal body, the anal canal and the perineal body.
B. **True.**
C. **True.**
D. **True.**
E. **False.** It contains the inferior rectal nerve and vessels, the labial (scrotal) nerve and vessels, the branch of the fourth sacral nerve and fat.

126.
A. **False.** The pituitary is entirely ectodermal in origin.
B. **False.** The pituitary lies in a depression in the sphenoid bone, the sella turcica.
C. **True.**
D. **True.** The pituitary is supplied with blood by the portal system originating in the hypothalamus (80%) and by a direct arterial supply.
E. **True.** Oxytocin and vasopressin are the two hormones produced by the posterior pituitary.

127.
A. **True.**
B. **True.** The continuation of the gubernaculum of the ovary is the round ligament which does reach the inguinal region.
C. **True.** The total number of germ cells rises from 600 000 at 2 months to a peak of 7 million at 5 months.
D. **False.** In early fetal life the ovaries lie in the lumbar region, near the kidney.
E. **True.** There is no peritoneal cover of the ovary in the adult.

128.
A. **True.**
B. **False.** Prolactin is the only hormone which is inhibited rather than stimulated by hypothalamic factors (dopamine).
C. **False.** The molecular weight is 24 000 daltons.
D. **True.** There is circadian variation, with high levels in the first part of the night.
E. **False.** It is produced by the acidophil cells of the anterior lobe of the pituitary gland, and its secretion is under the control of a hypothalamic inhibiting factor (dopamine).

129.

A. **False.** It is a protein hormone with no carbohydrate residues.
B. **False.** GH during pregnancy is not increased, and may actually be reduced because of the increased level of human placental lactogen (hPL).
C. **False.** Not for growth in the fetus.
D. **True.** GH secretion is reduced by medroxyprogestrone, rapid eye movement sleep, glucose, free fatty acids and cortisol.
E. **False.** GH is normal in pygmies, but insulin growth factor levels are low.

130.

A. **True.**
B. **True.**
C. **False.** The main control of aldosterone secretion is via the renin-angiotensin system.
D. **True.**
E. **True.** The remainder of the molecule (amino acids 18–39) is the corticotrophin-like intermediate lobe peptide (CLIP).

131.

A. **False.** It lies below and in front of the optic chiasma.
B. **False.** Vasopressin and oxytocin are released from the posterior pituitary gland.
C. **True.**
D. **True.**
E. **False.** The anterior pituitary is activated through the hypophyseal portal venous system.

132.

A. **True.**
B. **False.** Secretion is increased with sexual intercourse.
C. **True.** A glycosylated form of prolactin is secreted by the endometrium in the luteal phase of the cycle, and by the decidua in pregnancy.
D. **True.** Prolactin is secreted in the middle trimester of pregnancy, and increases progressively towards term.
E. **True.** The half-life is 6 h.

133.

A. **False.** Oxytocin is secreted by the paraventricular nuclei of the hypothalamus and stored in the posterior pituitary.
B. **False.** Alcohol inhibits the secretion of oxytocin and, in the past, has been used as a tocolytic to reduce uterine contractions in preterm labour.
C. **False.** Oxytocin has nine amino acids.
D. **True.** The uterus in early pregnancy is not very sensitive to oxytocin, but the latter may be used as a synergistic agent (with prostaglandin) in therapeutic abortion.
E. **True.** Hence, if used in a very dilute solution in labour, there is a risk of water intoxication and hyponatraemia.

134.
A. **True.** It lies in a depression in the sphenoid, the sella turcica, which is covered by a layer of dura mater (the diaphragma sellae) through which the pituitary stalk passes.
B. **True.**
C. **False.**
D. **True.** Its weight increases by 30–50 per cent due to an increase in prolactin-secreting cells.
E. **True.** Basophilic cells secrete thyroid-stimulating hormone (TSH), luteinizing hormone (LH), follicle-stimulating hormone (FSH) and pro-opiomelanocortin.

135.
A. **True.**
B. **False.** The hypothalamus forms part of the fore-brain.
C. **True.**
D. **False.** The hypothalamus regulates the activity of the anterior pituitary through the release of factors which are carried by veins of the pituitary stalk.
E. **False.** The hypothalamus forms part of the floor of the third ventricle.

136.
A. **True.** It secretes releasing hormones as a series of pulses, and the release is determined by the frequency rather than the amplitude of these pulses.
B. **True.**
C. **False.** The link is between the hypothalamus and the anterior pituitary.
D. **True.**
E. **True.**

137.
A. **True.** It is secreted by the supra-optic nuclei of the hypothalamus.
B. **True.**
C. **False.** The effect on blood pressure is only evident in large doses.
D. **True.**
E. **False.** Deficiency of vasopressin causes the clinical picture of diabetes insipidus.

138.
A. **True.**
B. **False.** It releases oxytocin and vasopressin.
C. **False.**
D. **True.** The permeability of the distal tubule and collecting ducts to water is increased. Water reabsorption is therefore increased, and urine volume decreased.
E. **True.** It arises as a down-growth of the neuroectoderm of the floor of the midbrain.

139.
A. True.
B. False. The greater the secretion of endogenous releasing hormone, the greater is the response to exogenous releasing factors. For example, the response to thyrotrophin-releasing hormone (TRH) in thyrotoxicosis is less than normal, whereas in hypothyroidism it is greater.
C. True.
D. False. The true figure is 42 amino acids.
E. True.

140.
A. False. FSH, as with thyroid-stimulating hormone (TSH), human chorionic gonadotrophin (hCG) and luteinizing hormone (LH) are glycoproteins composed of two subunits, alpha and beta.
B. True. In FSH, the alpha chain consists of 92 amino acids and two carbohydrate chains; the beta chain contains 111 amino acids and two carbohydrate chains.
C. True. The same as for the LH receptors.
D. False. It is produced by the chromophil cells of the anterior lobe of the pituitary gland.
E. False. FSH is responsible for early development, whereas LH is responsible for final maturity.

141.
A. False. The half-life of FSH is about 170 min, and that of LH is about 20 min (in some texts it is stated as being 60 min).
B. True.
C. True.
D. False. It causes no change in LH, but increases FSH secretion which characterizes early puberty.
E. False. Excreted in increased amounts at the climacteric and the menopause.

142.
A. True. It is also responsible for final maturation of the ovarian follicles.
B. True.
C. False. It has an initial flare-up effect (increased production of LH and FSH) followed by down-regulation (decreased production of LH and FSH).
D. False. The highest frequency is during the late luteal phase.
E. False. The highest amplitude is during the early luteal phase.

LH pulse frequency:

- Early follicular phase: 90 min
- Late follicular phase: 60–70 min
- Early luteal phase: 100 min
- Late luteal phase: 200 min

LH pulse amplitude:

- Early follicular phase: 6.5 IU/L
- Midfollicular phase: 5.0 IU/L
- Late follicular phase: 7.2 IU/L
- Early luteal phase: 15.0 IU/L
- Midluteal phase: 12.2 IU/L
- Late luteal phase: 8.0 IU/L

From Seifer, D.B. and Speroff, L. (1999).

143.
A. **True.** The higher content of sialic acid in FSH compared with LH accounts for the more rapid clearance of LH from the circulation (the FSH half-life is several hours; that of LH is about 20 min).
B. **True.**
C. **False.** The alpha chain is similar in the mentioned hormones, but the beta chain is unique in all hormones, conferring most of the specific functional properties of each hormone.
D. **True.**
E. **True.**

144.
A. **True.** Pregnancy and oestrogen administration also increase SHBG levels, whereas corticoids, androgens, progestins, growth hormone, insulin and insulin growth factor (IGF-1) decrease SHBG.
B. **False.** The majority are bound to a protein carrier, known as SHBG, that is produced in the liver. Another 10–30 per cent is loosely bound to albumin, leaving only about 1 per cent unbound and free. A very small percentage also binds to corticosteroid-binding globulin.
C. **False.** It occurs in the inner mitochondrial membrane.
D. **True.**
E. **True.**

Sex hormone	Free (unbound) (%)	Albumin-bound (%)	SHBG-bound (%)
Oestrogen	1	30	69
Testosterone	1	30	69
DHEA	4	88	8
Androstenedione	7	85	8
Dihydrotestosterone	1	71	28

DHEA = dihydroepiandrosterone.
From Seifer, D.B. and Speroff, L. (1999).

145.
A. **False.** Regular menstruation does not necessarily indicate regular ovulation.
B. **True.**
C. **True.**
D. **False.** The evidence is only fairly reliable.
E. **False.** Ovulation is unlikely up to 70 days in lactating women, and on average 45 days after delivery in non-lactating women.

146.
A. **False.** It occurs 12 h after the luteinizing hormone (LH) peak.
B. **True.**
C. **False.** Ferning is evidence that ovulation has occurred.
D. **False.** Ovum release takes about 2 min.
E. **True.**

147.
A. **False.** It develops in the gonadal ridge after 7 weeks' gestation.
B. **True.**
C. **False.** Mitotic proliferation produces large numbers of cells. It is the second meiotic division that generates genetic diversity and halves the chromosome number, and the third cytodifferentiation packages the chromosomes for effective delivery.
D. **False.** They descend through the inguinal canal in the third trimester (probably under the influence of androgens).
E. **False.** It requires not only the presence of the *SRY* gene but also its interaction with other genes.

> • The factor that determines whether the indifferent gonad will become a testis is called, appropriately, the testes-determining factor (TDF), a product of the Y chromosome.
>
> • The candidate for the TDF gene is located within a region named SRY, the sex-determining region of the Y chromosome.
>
> From Seifer, D.B. and Speroff, L. (1999).

148.
A. **False.** The peak is between 15 and 18 weeks, after which synthesis declines.
B. **False.** Sperm are stored in the vas deferens.
C. **False.** It depends on luteinizing hormone (LH).
D. **True.**
E. **True.** All mentioned hormones are secreted in small amounts, but the major portions of blood oestrone and oestradiol are derived by peripheral aromatization from blood androstenedione and testosterone, respectively.

149.
A. **True.** They remain as solid cords until a lumen forms at 4–5 years of age.
B. **True.**
C. **False.** Sperm are formed continuously from puberty. None can be found before puberty.
D. **True.** They have been found to still retain motility in the cervical canal and uterus for 5–7 days, and have been found in the tube 60 h after coitus. However, this does not mean they have the power to fertilize.
E. **True.** They are equivalent to granulosa cells in the ovary.

Normal values for semen analysis according to WHO:	
Volume	2.0 mL or more
Sperm concentration	20 million/mL or more
Motility	50% or more with forward progression, or 25% with rapid progression within 60 min of ejaculation
Morphology	30% or more normal forms
White blood cells	<1 million/mL
Immunobead test	<20% spermatozoa with adherent particles
SpermMar test	<10% spermatozoa with adherent particles

150.
A. **False.** Oestrogens have an 18-carbon-based nucleus.
B. **True.**
C. **False.** It is made up of one steroid binding unit and two non-binding subunits.
D. **False.** It is encoded on the short arm of chromosome 6.
E. **False.** FSH, luteinizing hormone (LH), human chorionic gonadotrophin (hCG) and thyroid-stimulating hormone (TSH) are all glycoproteins.

151.
A. **False.** The molecular weight is 4500 daltons.
B. **True.** They are synthesized on ribosomes and stored by the Golgi apparatus in separate vesicles within the same cell.
C. **True.** All steroids are bound to some extent to albumin. Some also have specific binding proteins in circulation. The binding to these proteins is of much higher affinity than to albumin, but their concentrations in plasma are less.
D. **True.**
E. **False.** hCG and LH act through the same receptor.

152.
A. **True.**
B. **False.** They are secreted by the adrenal cortex.
C. **False.** It is increased by oestradiol and decreased by testosterone.
D. **True.**
E. **True.**

153.
A. **True.**
B. **True.**
C. **False.** SHBG binds around 69 per cent of oestradiol in the blood, 30 per cent is bound to albumin, and 1 per cent is free and biologically active.
D. **False.** The principal oestrogen formed is oestriol, due to conversion of the fetal precursor 16-hydroxy-dehydroepiandrosterone (16OH-DHEA) by the placenta. As fetal 16OH-DHEA is the principal substrate for the oestrogen, urinary oestriol excretion of the mother can be monitored as an index of the state of the fetus.
E. **True.**

154.
A. **False.** Pubic and axillary hair growth occurs primarily due to androgens.
B. **False.** It decreases blood and urine levels of calcium, but it increases the calcification of bone.
C. **True.**
D. **True.**
E. **False.**

155.
A. **True.** The secretion rate is 10 mg per day.
B. **False.** DHT is 100 times more potent than testosterone.
C. **True.** This is the precocious development of the secondary sex characteristics without testicular growth.
D. **True.** Also it is possibly controlled by pituitary adrenal androgen-stimulating hormone.
E. **True.**

156.
A. **True.** It is also responsible for development of the external genitalia.
B. **True.**
C. **True.**
D. **True.**
E. **False.** It inhibits SHBG secretion.

157.
A. **False.** It exerts inhibitory effects at both levels, decreasing GnRH pulsatile secretion and GnRH pituitary response.
B. **True.**
C. **True.** Production of GnRH has been identified at other sites such as in the placenta, ovary and other regions of the brain.
D. **True.** This is why in Kallmann's syndrome there is an association between an absence of GnRH and a defect in sense of smell.
E. **False.** They are administered by subcutaneous or intramuscular injections, as a nasal spray, as sustained release implants or as injections. Oral administration of GnRH agonists is not effective.

158.
A. **False.** It is a steroid hormone, a C-19 derivative.
B. **False.** Systemic administration inhibits spermatogenesis.
C. **False.**
D. **True.** These include the deepening of the voice, body hair and penile growth.
E. **False.** It is secreted from the adrenal cortex.

159.
A. **True.** The metabolic activity of T_3 is four-fold that of T_4, so that the biological activity *in vivo* is approximately equal.
B. **False.** Thyroid hormone increases oxygen dissociation rather than decreases it.
C. **True.**
D. **True.** Reverse T_3 is also increased in starvation and after major surgery.
E. **False.** It remains more or less unchanged.

Reverse T$_3$

- Some T$_4$ is converted to an inactive isomer of T$_3$, reverse T$_3$. T$_3$ is especially prominent in the fetus.

From Chard, T. (2001).

160.
A. True.
B. True.
C. False. It has a short half-life of 2–6 h.
D. True.
E. True. Norepinephrine (noradrenaline) is facilitatory, and dopamine inhibitory.

161.
A. False. It develops as a thickening of the floor of the pharynx.
B. True.
C. False. T$_4$ can be detected before 18 weeks' gestation.
D. True. TBG levels are elevated by oral oestrogen and oestrogen of pregnancy. Levels are depressed by glucocorticoids, androgens and the anti-oestrogen, danazol. Although the total amount of T$_4$ is increased in pregnancy the mother remains euthyroid because the amount of free T$_4$ remains the same.
E. True.

162.
A. True.
B. False. 2 per cent is free, 80 per cent is bound to albumin, and 18 per cent is bound to corticosteroid-binding globulin.
C. True.
D. False. They are both expressed by a single gene.
E. True. This probably occurs by progesterone blocking the action of aldosterone on the kidney.

163.
A. True. It is probably responsible for the rise in basal body temperature at the time of ovulation.
B. True. It also enhances the negative feedback effects of oestradiol; thus injections of oestradiol into women during the progesterone-dominant phase of the menstrual cycle (luteal phase) is not followed by an LH surge.
C. False. It is decreased by progestins at both the transcriptional and translational levels, and is induced by oestrogen at the transcriptional level.
D. False. Only inhibited until the last few weeks of pregnancy.
E. True.

164.
A. **False.** At 3 months before ovulation, approximately 300 follicles will be recruited for development, though only 30 become gonadotrophin-dependent.
B. **True.**
C. **True.** There is also a greater number of gap junctions.
D. **False.** The theca interna of the follicle is the primary source of circulating oestrogen.
E. **True.**

165.
A. **False.** It is the surge of LH affecting the advanced follicles in two ways. First, it causes terminal growth changes in both the follicle cells and the oocyte, which results in expulsion from the follicle at ovulation. Second, the whole endocrinology of the follicle changes for it to become a corpus luteum.
B. **True.**
C. **True.**
D. **False.** Mainly progesterone is produced.
E. **True.**

166.
A. **False.** They are located predominantly in the nucleus.
B. **False.** Chemically, hPL is 90 per cent similar to GH, but has only 3 per cent of its activity.
C. **True.**
D. **False.** In which the products of cells diffuse in the extracellular fluid to affect neighbouring cells that may be some distance away.
E. **True.** Thus, they present in lower concentration compared to cortisol and progesterone, the receptors of which have short half-lives.

Intercellular communication:

- Neural communication: in which neurotransmitters are released at synaptic junctions from nerve cells and act across a narrow synaptic cleft on a post-synaptic cell.

- Endocrine communication: in which hormones and growth factors reach cells via the circulating blood.

- Paracrine communication: in which the products of cells diffuse in the extracellular fluid to affect neighbouring cells that may be some distance away.

From Ganong, W.F. (2001).

167.

A. **False.** They may cause this damage in the second/third trimester.
B. **True.** This occurs mainly in the third trimester.
C. **False.** Discoloration may occur in the second/third trimester.
D. **True.**
E. **True.**

168.

A. **True.**
B. **True.** Streptomycin is excreted unchanged by the kidney.
C. **False.** They are broad-spectrum antibiotics which are inactive against anaerobes.
D. **True.** It may also cause oral contraceptive failure.
E. **False.** It is similar, but not identical.

169.

A. **True.**
B. **True.**
C. **True.** Chloramphenicol is effective against common organisms as well as salmonella and rickettsiae.
D. **True.** But it is stable to lactamase.
E. **True.** Used in combination with metronidazole, this forms an effective regimen for the treatment of pelvic inflammatory disease.

170.

A. **False.** It only reduces the HIV-related mortality rate and the incidence and severity of opportunistic infections.
B. **False.** It enhances T-cell response.
C. **False.** Alpha-interferon is present in amniotic fluid and in the placenta.
D. **True.** Acyclovir itself is inactive. However, it is metabolized by a herpes simplex-specified enzyme (thymidine kinase) to cyclovir triphosphate, which prevents further DNA synthesis.
E. **True.**

171.

A. **False.** It is effective against influenza.
B. **False.** Its effect is only on cells containing the herpes virus; it does not prevent recurrence.
C. **True.** Alpha-interferon is produced by unstimulated T cells and monocytes. Beta-interferon is produced by stimulated epithelial cells in infected organs and by fibroblasts in tissue culture. Gamma-interferon is produced by sensitized T cells.
D. **True.**
E. **False.** It is too toxic for sytemic use.

172.

A. **True.**
B. **False.** Total dose not to be exceeded is 500 μg. It is essential not to exceed a concentration of 1 in 200 000 (5 μg/mL).
C. **True.** Thereby limiting transplacental exchange.
D. **True.**
E. **False.** It does not cause vasodilatation and is used in spinal anaesthesia.

173.

A. **True.**
B. **False.** It is rarely caused after extended use.
C. **False.** It is contra-indicated.
D. **True.**
E. **True.** It is an excellent induction agent. It has a narrow therapeutic margin, so cardiorespiratory depression may occur. It is also highly alkaline and therefore severely irritant if extravasated into tissues.

174.

A. **True.** It is usually used at a strength of 0.25 per cent, although higher concentrations may be used.
B. **False.** It is contra-indicated in ante-partum haemorrhage due to the dual risk of hypotension, but is useful in the management of pre-eclampsia.
C. **True.** If the spinal block rises to too high a level.
D. **True.** Due to relaxation of the levator ani it takes longer for the fetal head to descend and rotate after full dilatation.
E. **False.**

175.

A. **False.** The tricyclics prevent noradrenaline re-uptake by the nerve cells.
B. **True.**
C. **True.** If taken in the third trimester (especially imipramine).
D. **False.** They are effective in the treatment of moderate and severe degrees of depression.
E. **True.** Mainly in children.

176.

A. **True.** Arrhythmias and heart block occasionally follow tricyclic antidepressants, particularly amitriptyline.
B. **False.** It is not recommended, as safety and efficacy have not been established.
C. **True.** Tricyclic antidepressants have central and peripheral antimuscarinic actions.
D. **True.**
E. **True.**

177.
A. **True.**   They may provoke lactic acidosis.
B. **True.**   Biguanides only work in the presence of endogenous insulin, so there must be some residual islet cell function.
C. **False.**   Insulin is a polypeptide hormone of complex structure.
D. **False.**   Sulphonylureas do cross the placenta, and may result in fetal beta-cell stimulation.
E. **False.**   Insulin is bound to a beta-globulin.

178.
A. **True.**
B. **False.**   Glucagon, a polypeptide hormone produced by the alpha cells of the islets of Langerhans, increases mobilization of glycogen stored in the liver.
C. **False.**   Adrenaline activates the enzyme adenyl cyclase and leads to the formation of $3',5'$-cyclic adenosine monophosphate. This activates the enzyme phosphorylase kinase, which in turn catalyses the conversion of inactive to active phosphorylase. The latter effect leads to the breakdown of liver glycogen.
D. **True.**   Therefore it must be given by injection; the subcutaneous route is ideal in most circumstances
E. **False.**   Glucose and/or glucagon can be used in the treatment of hypoglycaemic coma. Glucagon is not effective for chronic hypoglycaemia.

179.
A. **True.**   PTU also inhibits coupling of iodotyrosines.
B. **True.**
C. **True.**
D. **True.**
E. **False.**   Intravenous liothyronine is the treatment of choice in hypothyroid coma.

180.
A. **False.**   TSH is synthetized and released from the anterior pituitary, and stimulates the release of thyroxine from the thyroid gland.
B. **True.**   As well as carbimazole, so the lowest effective dose is used.
C. **True.**
D. **False.**   Is not contra-indicated as the lowest dose that will control the thyroid should be used.
E. **True.**   The placenta is freely permeable to iodine and medications used to treat hyperthyroidism, such as propranolol, PTU and methimazole.

181.
A. **True.**
B. **False.**   Warfarin can cause nasal hypoplasia, chondrodysplasia punctata and CNS abnormalities. Gastroschisis is a recognized effect of pseudoephedrine.
C. **True.**
D. **True.**
E. **True.**

182.
A. True.
B. False. The femoral nerve appears at the lateral border of psoas, runs downward in the angle between iliacus and psoas, but does not enter the femoral sheath.
C. False. The inferior epigastric artery arises from the external iliac artery.
D. True.
E. False. The external iliac artery gives off the inferior epigastric and deep circumflex iliac branches before it passes under the inguinal ligament to become the femoral artery.

183.
A. True.
B. False. Its upper opening is referred to as the femoral ring.
C. True.
D. False. It contains one of the deep inguinal lymph nodes.
E. True. By the adherence of its medial wall to the tunica adventitia of the femoral vein.

184.
A. False.
B. True. Causes carcinoma of the vagina in young women, and vaginal adenosis.
C. True. Causes blindness and deafness.
D. True. It includes minor craniofacial and digital abnormalities, cardiac defects and cleft lip/palate.
E. True. Cause phocomelia, which involves absence of the long bones of the upper and/or lower limbs, among other defects.

185.
A. True.
B. True. It may cause masculinization in the female infant or precocious development in the male infant.
C. False. Safe as only trace amounts are secreted in milk.
D. True.
E. False. It is a loop diuretic.

186.
A. False. Warfarin is a small molecule and readily crosses the placenta. The two most common features are nasal hypoplasia and stippling of epiphyses.
B. True.
C. False. It is true for chlorpropramide but not chlorpheniramine, which is safe.
D. False. They cause deafness.
E. False.

187.

A. **False.** Vinblastine (a vinca alkaloid) arrests cells in metaphase of mitosis.
B. **True.**
C. **False.** Peripheral neuritis is not a recognized complication of methotrexate therapy.
D. **True.**
E. **True.**

188.

A. **True.** As it has an immunosuppressive action.
B. **True.**
C. **True.**
D. **False.** It prevents normal pyrimidine insertion into DNA.
E. **False.**

189.

A. **True.**
B. **False.** It takes about 7 min to act on the uterus.
C. **False.** Water intoxication and hyponatraemia.
D. **False.** Ritodrine is a beta-2 agonist which suppresses myometrial activity and is used to treat preterm labour.
E. **False.** Vomiting is a common side effect.

190.

A. **True.** It produces a prolonged tonic uterine contraction with superimposed rapid clonic contractions.
B. **False.** It causes smooth muscle relaxation of blood vessels and will tend to lower the blood pressure.
C. **False.** Oxytocin is an octapeptide hormone.
D. **True.**
E. **True.**

191.

A. **True.**
B. **False.** It is not advised as it has been implicated in intra-uterine closure of the fetal ductus arteriosus.
C. **True.**
D. **True.**
E. **False.** Oxytocin is produced by the posterior pituitary gland.

192.

A. **False.** It is rapidly inactivated in the liver and gut.
B. **True.**
C. **False.** It is more effective up to 5 days after unprotected intercourse.
D. **False.**
E. **True.**

193.

A. **False.** It is reduced by liver enzyme inducers (rifampicin, griseofulvin and most anticonvulsants).

B. **False.** They reduce the risk.

C. **True.** By competing for androgen receptors.

D. **True.**

E. **False.** Cyproterone acetate is an anti-androgen used in the treatment of hirsutism.

194.

A. **True.** It is an abortifacient.

B. **False.** Cyproterone acetate suppresses adrenocortical function.

C. **False.** Thyroid-binding globulin plasma concentration is increased.

D. **True.**

E. **True.** Progestogens should not be used in patients with a history of liver tumours, severe liver impairment, breast or genital cancer, severe arterial disease or undiagnosed vaginal bleeding.

195.

A. **False.** The incidence of ovarian and endometrial cancer is reduced in users of the combined oral contraceptive pill.

B. **True.**

C. **True.** 20 μg in low-strength preparations; 30–40 μg in standard-strength; and 50 μg in high-strength.

D. **False.** Progesterone deficiency is not the primary cause.

E. **False.** Replacement after 3 years is recommended.

196.

A. **False.** Transient vasoconstriction occurs first, followed by a prolonged period of vasodilatation.

B. **True.** In acutely inflamed tissues the clear zone becomes occupied by white cells.

C. **False.** Acute, rather than chronic inflammation.

D. **True.**

E. **True.** Kinins cause contraction of smooth muscle and are involved in local and general pain mechanisms.

197.

A. **True.**

B. **True.**

C. **True.**

D. **True.**

E. **True.**

198.
A. True.
B. True.
C. True.
D. False.
E. False. Occlusions occur in small arteries.

199.
A. True. It also forms a barrier against bacterial invasion, and aids phagocytosis.
B. False. They cause contraction of smooth muscle.
C. True. Diphtheria is associated with a neutrophilia.
D. True. Prostacyclin (PGI_2), which is produced by the endothelial cells of the blood vessels, causes vasodilatation and increased capillary permeability.
E. False. The neutrophil polymorphs are the first cells to emigrate through the endothelial gaps in acute inflammation.

200.
A. False. The chancre is a very firm painless nodule which ulcerates and becomes very infectious.
B. True.
C. False. It is not specific; yaws, pinta and bejel give positive reactions.
D. False. It is a feature of tertiary syphilis.
E. True. The causative organism is *Treponema pallidum*, a delicate spiral filament which is about 10 μm in length.

201.
A. True.
B. True.
C. True.
D. True.
E. True.

202.
A. False. There is deposition of 'amyloid material' (complex mucopolysaccharide-containing globulins) in the connective tissue stroma and the walls of blood vessels of certain tissues and organs.
B. False.
C. True.
D. True.
E. False. The liver is enlarged, heavy, pale and firm.

203.
A. **False.** Siderocytes are red cells containing haemosiderin, and they are increased in number after excessive iron intake.
B. **False.** *Mycobacterium tuberculosis* is very resistant to drying.
C. **True.**
D. **False.** Until 1976, all strains were penicillin-sensitive, but since then increasing reports of beta-lactamase-producing, penicillin-resistant organisms have appeared.
E. **True.** Tuberculosis of the genital tract is almost always a blood-borne infection from a focus elsewhere (usually in the lungs).

204.
A. **True.**
B. **True.**
C. **True.** Histamine has a potent stimulatory effect on gastric acid secretion and is present in high concentrations in the gastric mucosa.
D. **False.** Acute inflammatory exudate contains fibrin: it clots readily on standing.
E. **False.** Serotonin is released from mast cells and plays a similar role to histamine.

205.
A. **True.** Wound healing is delayed by infection, steroid administration and external radiation.
B. **False.** Collagen is a protein providing structural integrity to tissues.
C. **False.** Nerve cells cannot divide or regenerate.
D. **True.**
E. **True.**

206.
A. **True.** Zinc deficiency impairs the strength of scars.
B. **False.** The demolition phase is followed by an acute inflammation phase.
C. **False.** Highly vascular areas such as the face and scalp heal faster than less vascular areas such as the trunk and limbs.
D. **False.** The limit is 1–2 cm.
E. **True.**

207.
A. **False.** Body fat is the main source of energy as it can yield up to 3000 calories per day versus a total of 1600 calories for liver glycogen.
B. **True.** It reaches up to 100–300 mmol in the first week.
C. **False.** Insulin secretion is reduced, so liver gluconeogenesis is promoted and this will contribute to the hyperglycaemia.
D. **False.** The specific gravity for the urine remains above 1.015, unless there is renal damage.
E. **True.** It is converted to glucose, pyruvate and lactate.

208.
A. **True.** Which promotes reabsorption of water from distal tubules.
B. **False.** Replacement of plasma proteins takes 2–3 days.
C. **True.** Nitrogen excretion is increased to 25 g per day.
D. **True.** Catecholamines have a lipolytic effect, so fatty acids are released from adipose tissues.
E. **True.** In addition to peripheral vasoconstriction, a rise in diastolic blood pressure and pulse rate, release of glucose and cortisol and quickening of reaction times.

209.
A. **False.** Shock is the clinical state in which the patient is tachycardic, pale and sweating.
B. **False.** Kidney damage in endotoxic shock is caused by direct damage to the renal epithelium, and also circulatory changes.
C. **True.**
D. **False.** Hypovolaemic shock follows haemorrhage of 20 per cent or more of blood volume. It may also be provoked by the excess fluid loss from burns.
E. **True.** There is a profound reduction in metabolic rate, the nature of which is not well understood.

210.
A. **True.** Massive doses of steroids may be helpful in reducing the passage of fluid and cells across the capillary walls.
B. **True.**
C. **True.** Hypovolaemic shock may follow gut infections such as cholera.
D. **True.**
E. **False.** Endotoxic shock is caused by lipopolysaccharide toxins.

211.
A. **True.**
B. **True.**
C. **False.** Herpes type II.
D. **False.** Carcinoma of cervix.
E. **False.** Hepatoma.

212.
A. **True.**
B. **True.**
C. **True.**
D. **True.**
E. **True.**

213.
A. True.
B. False. It is asymptomatic and detected only by cytological and/or colposcopic examination.
C. False. It is a cytological term. Dysplasia is a histological term and refers to abnormalities of tissues.
D. True.
E. False. 90 per cent.

214.
A. False. Skin and paraffin industry.
B. True.
C. True.
D. False. Woodworkers.
E. True.

215.
A. True.
B. False. It has low incidence in Japan.
C. False. It arises from embryonic elements and is commonest at age 20–45 years.
D. True.
E. False. Seminoma is a carcinoma of the testis derived from the seminiferous epithelium.

216.
A. False. Breast cancer is the commonest malignant growth, but affects only 1 per cent of men.
B. False. Carcinoma of the prostate usually occurs over the age of 60 years.
C. True.
D. True.
E. False. *Schistosoma haematobium* is associated with bladder cancer.

217.
A. False. Conn's tumour secretes aldosterone.
B. True. Pulmonary and cardiac effects are well documented.
C. True.
D. True. Dysgerminoma is very sensitive to radiotherapy.
E. False. Carcinoma of the prostate characteristically leads to osteosclerotic bone metastases.

218.
A. False.
B. True. It is a childhood tumour which arises from any type of connective tissue.
C. True. Is a malignant tumour of the spermatocytes.
D. False. Lipoma are benign tumours of fat cells.
E. False.

219.
A. True. This is Cushing's disease.
B. False. They produce alpha fetoprotein.
C. False. It produces catecholamines.
D. False. Carcinoids secrete 5-hydroxytryptamine.
E. True. They secret oestrogen in about two-thirds of patients presenting with abnormal vaginal bleeding.

220.
A. True.
B. True.
C. False. Melanin is produced from tyrosine.
D. False. It is a carcinoma derived from the seminiferous epithelium.
E. False. Acanthoma is a special form of squamous cell carcinoma. Acanthosis is a proliferation of the prickle-cell layer.

221.
A. False. Fast-growing tumours have a doubling time of 10–25 days.
B. False. This has only been shown in lymphomas and leukaemias.
C. False. Invasion of surrounding tissues is the characteristic feature of malignant tumours.
D. True. An example is cancer of the lip.
E. True. As well as massively increased.

222.
A. True.
B. False. Immunoglobulins G are produced by plasma cells.
C. False. The majority of immunoglobulins are gamma-globulins, but there is some electrophoretic activity in the alpha and beta regions.
D. False. Kappa light chains are coded for on chromosome 12, lambda chains on chromosome 22, and heavy chains on chromosome 14.
E. True.

223.
A. False. Babies do not start producing their own IgG until the maternal IgG has been catabolized at about 3–4 months of age.
B. False. Individuals vary widely in their production of IgG.
C. True.
D. True.
E. False. Complement is activated by many antigen–antibody reactions, but is not required for antibody formation.

224.
A. **False.** The basic immunoglobulin molecule consists of four peptide chains.
B. **False.** IgA plasma concentration is 200 mg/dL, while that of IgG is 1000 mg/dL.
C. **True.**
D. **False.** The activated B cells proliferate and transform into memory cells and plasma cells which secrete the antibodies.
E. **True.** This is important in affording the neonate passive immunity before its own immune system has matured.

225.
A. **True.** The two long chains are called heavy chains; the two short chains are called light chains.
B. **False.** The variable regions of one heavy chain and one light chain form an antigen-binding site.
C. **False.** Immunoglobulins are produced by B cells.
D. **True.** Also reagin activity.
E. **True.** Examples are intestinal fluids, saliva and bronchial secretions.

226.
A. **True.**
B. **True.**
C. **True.** Anti-Kell antibodies can cause haemolytic disease in babies born to rhesus positive or negative mothers. Thus, the baby should be treated in the same way as any baby born to a rhesus negative mother. Cord bloods are tested for haemoglobin, blood group, bilirubin and Coomb's test.
D. **False.** Maternal IgM levels are very low in the umbilical cord.
E. **True.**

227.
A. **True.**
B. **True.** In term infants, the plasma concentration of these factors is similar to normal adult values.
C. **False.** Platelet counts are normal.
D. **False.** Anti-Lewis antibodies are not haemolytic as the antigen is absorbed from the plasma and is not an intrinsic part of the red blood cell membrane.
E. **False.** An indirect Coombs' test detects the presence of free immunoglobin in the serum; a direct Coombs' test detects the presence of attached immunoglobulin in red blood cells.

228.
A. **True.**
B. **False.** There are reduced levels of T helper cells in normal pregnancy.
C. **False.** Occasionally, maternal IgG may be harmful to the fetus, as in rhesus isoimmunization or maternal immune thrombocytopenic purpura.
D. **False.** Maternal IgM does not cross the placenta in humans, but may do so in certain species.
E. **True.**

229.

A. **True.** It acts on macrophages to increase their ability to kill ingested bacteria and tumour cells.
B. **True.**
C. **False.** Also from other cells.
D. **True.**
E. **True.**

230.

A. **True.**
B. **True.**
C. **True.**
D. **True.** And released after lymphocytic stimulation.
E. **True.**

231.

A. **False.** It is C3.
B. **False.** They are soluble proteins.
C. **True.**
D. **False.** This is true for the classical pathway, while the alternative is activated by the action of microbial polysaccharides and aggregated IgA or IgG.
E. **True.** The amplification loop: C3Bb can itself become a C3 convertase, thus triggering more C3b formation. This causes amplification of both classical and alternative pathways.

232.

A. **False.** It comprises three morphologically and functionally distinct regions called the zona glomerulosa (the outer), zona fasiculata (the intermediate) and zona reticularis (the inner).
B. **False.** The fetal adrenal cortex represent 80 per cent of the gland which undergoes rapid regression at the time of birth.
C. **True.**
D. **False.** Zona fasciculata is the intermediate layer and it produces cortisol.
E. **False.** Because of the action of angiotensin II on the zona glomerulosa, it will remain unchanged.

233.

A. **True.**
B. **True.**
C. **False.** The upper part of the rectum is covered with peritoneum in front and at the sides, the middle part is covered in front only; the lower part lies below the level of the rectovaginal pouch and therefore is devoid of peritoneal covering.
D. **False.** Blood supply is from the inferior mesenteric artery through its rectal branches.
E. **False.** Appendices epiploicae and taenia coli are only found in association with the colon.

234.

A. **False.** The cutaneous lymph vessels above the umbilicus drain into the anterior axillary lymph nodes, while the vessels below this level drain into the superficial inguinal lymph nodes.

B. **True.**

C. **True.**

D. **False.** It heals as a wide or heaped-up scar. Incisions along the natural lines of cleavage heal better.

E. **True.** And also the pyramidalis muscle.

235.

A. **True.**

B. **False.** It lies in front of the anal canal, and behind the posterior border of the perineal membrane.

C. **True.** Bulbocavernosus, transverse perineal, external anal sphincter and levator ani muscles all insert into the perineal body.

D. **False.** It is a fibromuscular mass.

E. **False.** The puborectalis is part of the levator ani muscle and is therefore above the perineal body.

236.

A. **True.**

B. **True.**

C. **False.**

D. **True.**

E. **False.**

The female breast

- Extends from the 2nd to the 6th rib vertically, and from the parasternal margin to the midaxillary line horizontally.

- Consists of 15–25 lobes, each of which drains 20–40 lobules into which 10–100 alevoli drain.

- Arterial blood supply is from the internal mammary, lateral thoracic, intercostal and acromio-thoracic arteries.

- Venous return follows those arteries and is received in the large, mainly valveless veins that also drain the vertebrae.

- Breast malignancy spreads to the bodies of the vertebrae by reflux flow through these veins.

237.
A. True.
B. False. The vestibule lies between the hymen and the labia minora.
C. True.
D. True.
E. True.

238.
A. True.
B. True.
C. False. There is no fat beneath the skin of the areola and nipple.
D. True. In females, the breasts develop primarily under the control of oestrogens, which cause proliferation of the mammary ducts; and progesterone, which results in the development of the lobules.
E. False.

239.
A. False. The labia minora develop from the genital fold, while the labia majora develop from genital swellings.
B. True.
C. False. The epithelium is keratinized on the lateral side only.
D. False. The nerve endings are similar to, but less abundant than, those of the labia majora.
E. True. And also to the superficial inguinal nodes.

240.
A. True. It is created from Rathke's pouch, an upward evagination of the ectoderm of the pharyngeal roof.
B. True. By 30–50 per cent due to an increase in the secretion of prolactin.
C. False. There are no releasing factors produced.
D. False. Basophil cells secrete thyroid-stimulating hormone (TSH), follicle-stimulating hormone (FSH), ACTH and its precursor (pro-opiocortin).
E. True. It is supplied by the portal system originating from the hypothalamus (80%), and by a direct arterial supply.

Bibliography

Chamberlain, G., Broughton Pipkin, F. *Clinical Physiology in Obstetrics*. 3rd edition. Blackwell Science, Oxford, 1998.

Chard, T. *Basic Sciences for Obstetrics and Gynaecology MCQs*. 2nd edition. Springer

Edmonds D.K. (ed.) *Dewhurst's Textboook of Obstetrics and Gynaecology for Postgraduates*. 6th edition. Blackwell Science, London, 1998.

Frederickson, H. and Wilkins-Haug, L. *Ob/Gyn Secrets*. 2nd edition. Hanley & Belfus, Philadelphia, 1997.

Ganong, W.F. *Review of Medical Physiology*. 20th edition. McGraw Hill, New York, 2001.

Johnson, M., Everitt, B.J. *Essential Reproduction*. 5th edition. Blackwell Science, Oxford, 1999.

Kingston, H.M. *ABC of Clinical Genetics*. 2nd edition. BMJ, London, 1997.

Sadler, T.W. *Langman's Medical Embryology*. 8th edition. Lippincott, Williams & Wilkins, Philadelphia, 2000.

Seiffer, D.B. and Sperof, L. (eds) *Clinical Gynecologic Endocrinology and Infertility*. 6th edition. Lippincott, Williams & Wilkins, Philadelphia,1999.

Snell, R.S. *Clinical Anatomy for Medical Students*. 6th edition. Little, Brown and Company, London, 2000.

De Swiet, M., Chamberlain, G., Bennett, P. *Basic Science in Obstetrics and Gynaecology. A Textbook for MRCOG Part 1*. Churchill Livingstone, London, 2001.

Veralls, S. *Anatomy and Physiology Applied to Obstetrics*. 3rd edition. Churchill Livingstone, London, 1993.

Walter, J.B., and Grundy, M.C. *Walter, Hamilton and Israel's Principles of Pathology for Dental Students*. 5th edition. Churchill Livingstone, London, 1992.

Index

Using the self-assessment CD-ROM

This CD will work on all PC systems, except for Windows 2000 Professional

To install the program:

- Double-click on the CD-ROM icon on your computer to open the CD.
- Double-click on the 'setup' application.
- The install program will run. Follow the instructions on screen.
- You can choose where the program will be installed on your system. The default will usually be C:\Programfiles, but you can alter this if you wish. Remember where you have installed the program.
- Once the install is complete, you can remove the CD from the drive. You will not need to insert the CD again, unless at some point you uninstall the files from your system, and need to install them again.

To run the program:

- Run the program by double-clicking on the 'MCQ' icon in the Program Files folder on your C-Drive (or the place where you installed the files, if not in Program Files).
- You have one hour to complete 30 multi-stem MCQs.
- Tick the boxes to the right of the screen: T = true, F = false, DK = don't know.
- At the bottom of the screen, click   > to go forward to the next question

                               < to go back to the previous question

                               >> to go to the last question in the test

                               << to go back to the first question
- Click 'finish' at any time to see the answers, you do not have to wait until you have completed all 30 questions. The program then goes into 'Revision mode'.
- Again, use the direction buttons at the bottom of the screen to see how you did on each MCQ.
- Red = an incorrect answer (also shown by a cross symbol).
- Green = a correct answer (also shown by a tick symbol).
- A yellow bullet next to the question letter indicates that further information is available. Click on the question text to get this information, then click on 'OK' to return to the main screen.
- Click 'Report' to get a breakdown of your scores.